PENGUIN BOOKS
HOME REMEDIES
VOLUME TWO

T. V. Sairam, a senior member of the civil services, holds a Master's degree in botany and a doctorate in alternative medicine. For the past three decades he has been gathering and documenting data relating to the household use of medicinal plants.

'The book presents the material related to 40 common medicinal plants . . . in a very lucid manner . . . The most useful part of the book is that it provides notes on preparation of herbal medicine, dosage and some thumb rules for the selection of the various parts of the medicinal plant. . . . An interesting bibliography also accompanies the book . . . a complete guide on medicinal herbs. It caters to the need of both the common man and a practitioner alike.'
—*Deccan Herald*

'. . . an excellent and beautifully produced book, rich in information . . . The chapters have been structured thoughtfully . . . The author has produced an eminently readable and useful book . . .'
—*Indian Review of Books*

'The author meticulously documents many parallel traditions and their uses of individual plants to cure and comfort . . . an illuminating rediscovery of herbs . . .'
—*First City*

'A glossary of English medical terms and the Indian names of the herbs in quite a few regional languages does prove helpful.'
—*The Statesman*

'Years of research on ancient herblore by T.V. Sairam is slowly but surely taking the shape of easy-to-use volumes on the medicinal values of the phenomenal wealth the country has in herbs . . .'
—*The Hindu*

'A very useful book.'
—*The Financial Express*

Home Remedies Volume Two

A Handbook of Herbal Cures for Common Ailments

T. V. SAIRAM

Illustrations by Amitabh

PENGUIN BOOKS

An imprint of Penguin Random House

PENGUIN BOOKS

USA | Canada | UK | Ireland | Australia
New Zealand | India | South Africa | China | Singapore

Penguin Books is part of the Penguin Random House group of companies
whose addresses can be found at global.penguinrandomhouse.com

Published by Penguin Random House India Pvt. Ltd
4th Floor, Capital Tower 1, MG Road,
Gurugram 122 002, Haryana, India

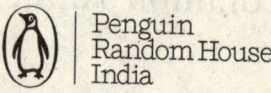

First published by Penguin Books India 1999

While every effort has been made to verify the authenticity of the information
contained in this book, it is not intended as a substitute for medical consultation
with a physician. The publisher and the author are in no way liable for the use of
the information contained in the book.

ISBN 9780140288186

Typeset in Adobe Garamond by Eleven Arts, New Delhi
Printed at Repro India Limited

www.penguin.co.in

This is a legitimate digitally printed version of the book and therefore might not
have certain extra finishing on the cover.

For the innumerable
housewives, ojhas, hakims and vaidyars
who continue to practise their
arts in difficult times

Contents

CONTENTS

Preface

Systematic research in various systems of Indian medicine under the patronage of the Government of India commenced in the year 1969 with the establishment of the Central Council for Research in Indian Medicine and Homoeopathy (CCRIMH). In 1978, this body was split into four separate research councils: one each for Ayurveda and Siddha, Unani medicine, Homoeopathy, and Yoga and Naturopathy.

A recent WHO estimate reveals that around 80 per cent of the global population consume phyto-medicines, and documents a shift in emphasis from the underdeveloped to the developed countries of the world. This trend has both positive and negative fallouts in society. While the prices of useful herbs skyrocket in the developing world as their main sources are depleted, the rural poor who have long been dependent on them find them unaffordable when compared to synthetic drugs and medicines. Even in the remote corners of rural and tribal India, we notice that branded synthetic medicines manufactured by multinational concerns have begun to percolate.

A survey conducted by researchers at the Beth Israel Deaconess Medical Centre and the Harvard Medical School in Boston reveals that the use of herbal medicines and other alternative therapies has shown a steep rise in the United States, with sales of herbal remedies increasing by 380 per cent during the nineties. The number of visits made by American patients to herbalists, chiropractors and other purveyors of alternative medicine is reported to exceed the total visits to all primary-care physicians.

The trend indicates the changing attitudes in modern society in general with regard to complementary and alternative systems of medicine.

A comparative study of ethno-botanical information contained in ancient Indian literature with folk medical lore, research amongst tribal communities and current scientific findings can go a long way in establishing the direction of future medical exploration.

The recent publication of the *Indian Herbal Pharmacopoeia* is a giant leap in this direction; some herbs have been standardized and twenty herbs have had monographs devoted to them. No doubt much work remains to be done. In order to obtain consistent results, the standardization of the product has to be monitored right from the raw-material stage. The habitat of the plant and the time of collection play a vital role in achieving consistency.

Although there have been attempts at a broader understanding of drugs based on their chemistry and pharmacology, India can perhaps follow China, where experimental results are immediately passed on to clinical investigators, who provide the necessary support in the clinical evaluation of particular drugs.

The Indian subcontinent contains about 25,000 species of vascular plants, of which 7500 are used by folk and other traditional systems of medicine. Many plants are common to all the traditional systems. Several are used either alone or in combination with other plants. The current regulations state that if these drugs are prepared in exactly the same way as laid down in ancient literature and if they are preserved as detailed by the texts, such drugs do not require either approval of registration. The drug will however be treated as 'new' whenever a different method of preparation is used.

The subcontinent occupies a unique position in the world, capable of cultivating most of the medicinal plants used both in modern as well as traditional systems of medicine.

While India has to travel a long way to become self-sufficient in pharmaceutical production, the largest chunk of medicines—almost 70 per cent—draw on the indigenous systems of medicine catering to the needs of most of our rural people.

The export value of crude drugs from India in the international market has increased 2.76 times between 1985–86 and 1994–95, and now stands at 53.2 million.

Although India is one of the major suppliers of medicinal plants to the world, the export of value-added materials such as plant derivatives, chemicals, etc. is insignificant compared to the developed countries.

According to an UNIDO study, although there were 3349 units licensed to manufacture plant-based pharmaceuticals in 1987, their contribution to the total production was considered marginal.

A systematic survey of all medicinal flora is the need of the hour. While that may safely be left to dedicated researchers, this book is my attempt to contribute by documenting and making available to a larger public what I have seen practised in the course of my researches.

This second volume of *Home Remedies* follows on from where the first had left off, hoping to reclaim a place on our kitchen shelves and in our lives for plants we have come to dismiss lightly.

Introduction

> *For cutting off the tender sprouts, a fine of six*
> *panas will be imposed; for cutting off the minor*
> *branches, twelve panas and for cutting off the big*
> *branches, twenty-four panas. Cutting off the trunk*
> *will be punished with the first amercement; and*
> *felling will be punished with the middlemost*
> *amercement.*

—Arthashastra, III 19:197

The writing of this book was undertaken to fill what I perceive to be a serious void between the ethnic discovery of herbs and their scientific rediscovery.

It was felt that collecting and categorizing available data from folklore as well as the Western scientific literature on medicinal herbs would facilitate an informed understanding that could better evaluate the premises and methodology of the complicated and often misunderstood role of herbalism and alternative medicine. Herbs are often seen as the last resort once all other avenues of treatment have been exhausted. Being approached as last-minute miracle workers serves to reinforce the mystic aura associated with such systems of medicine, thus discounting the sophisticated and ancient herb lore that its practitioners draw on. The hereditary household remedial system handed down by often unlettered women, the village vaids, hakims and ojhas and their travelling counterparts represent the fragmentary remnants of systems evolved to perfection to meet the needs of localized communities, drawing on familiar plants and locally available materials to treat ailments. Such practices are however fast becoming extinct, and I have often noted on my travels that even in a far-flung village, it has become the fashion to go for a tablet of aspirin rather than a piece of ginger, unmindful of the feeble voice of a family elder or the village physician.

Systematic documentation of this knowledge becomes an urgent necessity in the face of such onslaughts, as has been made clear to me time and again on my frequent trips to remote areas. The Kotas, among one of the ancient inhabitants of the Nilgiris, have all but lost their familiarity with their native medicines. Their villages which till recently boasted of a village physician, now totally depend on the nearby hospitals for treating even the simplest of ailments.

An identical situation prevails in a village near Hyderabad. Almost the entire village was suffering from malnutrition due to vitamin deficiency. The villagers squarely blamed the government for their plight and pointed out that the local dispensaries never maintained adequate stocks of vitamins. All this was in spite of the surprisingly large number of drumstick trees which were growing almost everywhere in the village! All the vitamin-loaded leaves of the trees were ironically ending up as manure or cattle feed.

The ancient methods designed for optimum beneficial use of local resources are in danger in ways that classical systems such as Ayurveda, Unani and Siddha have overcome. These classical systems have been elaborately documented in the form of verses, which survive as manuscripts in the written form, or are passed on from generation to generation orally. Herbal folklore however continues to be unrecorded and as a consequence, endangered.

India has always been a treasure trove of herbs. Historically in traditional Indian cuisine, there was hardly any distinction between food and medicine. Herbs were seen as agents of satisfaction and well being. Centuries before the birth of the

Greek and Roman empires, Indian ships carried herbs and their derivatives like perfumes and textiles to far-off destinations like Arabia, Mesopotamia and Egypt. The subcontinent's wealth of flora derives from the wide variations in geo-climactic and ecological endowments—tropical, temperate, alpine and arid zones, fluctuating factors such as relative humidity, temperature, monsoon, etc. The sheer variety of herbs and spices available to early shamans and physicians and their rich herb mythology and herb lore lured human migration not only from her neighbourhood but also from distant lands.

Later, it was Indian spices that wrote a fascinating history of adventure, exploration, conquest and colonialism. Bitter sea battles were fought over the spice growing colonies. The treasures of herbs and spices have always been indicators of wealth and status and have dictated the policies of nations. Indian herbalism was developed by the ancient seers, sages, wanderers and tribals who through intuition and observation discovered the many properties of plants and their products. The wisdom and experience of generations was consolidated in its growth. Over the millenia, other herbal systems and herbs brought into the subcontinent grew and added to indigenous lore.

Today it is easy to forget that the original sources of modern medicine were unsung folk prescriptions: morphine from poppy, quinine from cinchona, ephedrine from ma-huang, digitalin from foxglove. Today too, there are people who still treat minor ailments inexpensively with remedies taught to them by their forebears. This is especially true of folk medicine and simple home remedies and beauty aids taught to young girls by their grandmothers in many parts of the country. The body of information accumulated in these and other systems of medicine, dealing with the specific medicinal applications of herbs for specific complaints, has been tested innumerable times over the millenia in actual practice.

Scientific Interest in Herbs

The term herb technically refers to a non-woody plant that dies down to the ground after flowering. In general use, it refers to any plant species, including trees. Plants are the chemical factories of nature. The spectacular progress in organic chemistry has rendered most of the natural products amenable to synthesis. In the late eighteenth century and the nineteenth century, organic chemists occupied centre-stage. Recognizing the importance of plant materials, they isolated the active ingredients of many plants and plant products—nimbidin from *Azadirachta indica* (Neem), hyosine from *Datura metel* (Green Thorn Apple), and reserpine from *Rauwolfia serpentina* (Sarpagandha). In the twentieth century, the sixties saw the phytochemists working with randomly chosen plants. In the seventies growing interest in folkloric drugs urged these qualified researchers to select and work on plants used in traditional medicine. In the eighties and nineties these studies, aimed at the isolation and structure elucidation of the chemical constituents of the chosen plants, were pursued further. Despite such investigation, it is estimated that ninety per cent of recorded flora remains unstudied. However, the ultimate aim of scientific interest in traditional drugs is neither to ascribe them formal recognition or to explore their use as just alternatives or supplements to modern medicine.

The medical recipes and therapies gathered by me from diverse sources deserve very serious and urgent consideration by scientific and medical researchers. I think the time has come for the scientific community not to rest content with the isolation of 'active principles' alone from these plants. This 'classical' approach by scientists seeking to pinpoint single active substances and either extract them as they are or synthesize them in the laboratories serves only a limited purpose, since we are already aware that plants also contain secondary enhancing and/or side-effect-eliminating substances, which are lost for good in the process of isolation of active principles. Besides, there is greater scope for researchers to discover which chemical appears in which part of the plant and when. Apart from verifying existing scientific findings and explaining the role of plants in modern biochemical terms, which I understand that the Herb Society in London has currently undertaken, there is a need for a scientific understanding of systems of alternative medicine that have proved useful for suffering humanity, and for which no scientific explanation has yet emerged. The scientific community by transcending its mindset would perhaps be able to find a satisfactory answer to this in the coming years.

Herbalism in India is today beset by myriad problems. The value of the medicinal plant depends on its active principle content and not on its abundant growth or harvest. This aspect distinguishes the herbal industry from the others as the norms of production of agricultural crops differ.

Moreover, it is often found that the same plant grown in different localities differs widely in its medicinal value. Several factors such as soil, rainfall, latitude, altitude, method of cultivation, time of collection, storage, transport, etc play an important role in the medicinal value of drugs.

A wholesome and uniform *Materia Medica* appears a distant dream even today.

What is worse, there is no attempt to identify correct plant species mentioned in various vernacular literatures. There is also no serious attempt to document even today all available information on herbs mentioned in the vernacular treatises lying scattered over the length and breadth of the country, or to confirm and consolidate information relating to the affective part of the plant or its dosage and the application-methodology, particularly the details relating to combining the herbs.

Although most of the vernacular treatises make an attempt to broadly communicate the uses of plants, there is little other detail in them, meant as they are for the expert practising physician. Particulars such as exact dosage, duration of treatment, etc are often left to the imagination of the lay and often unlettered present-day practitioners. There is thus a need for formulating the effective dosage and treatment-duration in respect of each herb/herbal product.

There is also widespread practice of substitution of herbs and ingredients. This is a very serious offence which unfortunately goes unnoticed or un-reported. It is necessary that some institutional checks are initiated with a view to ensure purity and quality of herbal products.

I can find no better way to end, than with this beautiful story that emphasizes the need to preserve our ancient skills. The story tells of the legendary Jivaka, who was the royal physician during Buddha's time.

On completion of his seven-year medical course at Taxila, Jivaka was given the following problem by the examiner: 'Take this spade and seek around Taxila, a yojana on every side and whatever plant you see which is not medicinal, bring it to me.'

Jivaka, so the legend goes, examined all the plants in the specified area and was forced to return to the examiner empty-handed!

How to Use the Book

The book deals with forty commonly found herbs in the subcontinent, some of them familiar kitchen and spice box staples that are invariably accompanied by some minimal knowledge of their therapeutic properties, even in urban homes. The majority of these herbs are indigenous, though some were brought into the country by incoming invaders, colonisers and migrants. Over a period of time, they have merged so much with Indian gastronomy and medicine that their place of origin appears to be irrelevant. While dealing with each herb, I have recorded its traditional use along with recent scientific information, particularly its efficacy as a drug. A list of references from scientific research work indicating the composition and efficacy of herbs and their constituents will enable each reader to arrive at his or her own evaluation of the relevance of both the traditional practices and the scientific literature. The *In Tradition* pages record the accepted remedies for specific ailments that draw upon each herb's unique therapeutic properties. The ailments are arranged in alphabetical order, as usually classified in medical terminology.

While each entry has been alphabetized, certain groups of related symptoms that cover more than one system have not been separated, since all or a few of them may occur simultaneously. The extensive index at the back of the book allows quick location of multiple remedies for the same ailment, and a choice of herbs. The intuitive preference of certain herbs over others is the best pointer in choosing the appropriate remedy. As many Indian language names as possible have been recorded, thus enabling easy identification of the herbs. The multi language index facilitates the location of herbs by their familiar names, rather than the botanical or English ones. The detailed line drawings that accompany each herb further underline their familiarity while linking us to forgotten healing traditions.

The book records traditional medicinal remedies that are in danger of falling into disuse in forms in which they have been handed down across generations of practitioners. Traditional household practises regarding dosage, application and combination of herbs for alleviating symptoms and curing ailments were all gathered by me mostly through word of mouth from hundreds of housewives, illiterate grandmothers, vaids and ojhas, who voluntarily came forward to reveal them, including specialized tips derived from a lifetime of experience. These living herbals of folk usage will hopefully be the starting points for a comprehensive *Herbal Materia Medica*. Tips on certain herbal preparations that serve as inexpensive substitutes for their chemical-based brethren in the markets are included wherever possible. A comprehensive medical and herbal glossary and one of Non-English terms explains technical concepts from various systems of medicine.

Herbal Preparations: Some Guidelines

There could be some confusion regarding the preparation of home remedies for lay readers. An attempt is made here to explain the various procedures, processes and preparations dealt with in this book.

Notes on Preparation

In traditional systems of medicine, particularly the ones prevalent in South India, one often comes across the practice of mixing honey with almost every herbal powder or *bhasma,* etc. Honey is regarded as an essential vehicle that aids easy digestion and assimilation of the drug. Whenever honey is not available, other sweet substances such as jaggery, sugar candy, etc are powdered and mixed with the drug. As in Ayurveda, balancing of tastes is an important phenomenon and drugs which are bitter, sour or astringent are often mixed with sweet substances and administered.

Resins and Gums. Resins and gums exude from the branches of several trees, especially *Acacia.* They are generally harvested in the dry seasons, by making wounds on their branches and trunks. The liquid exudate which solidifies quickly is then scraped off the tree with the help of a knife. In the case of myrrh (*Commiphora myrrha*), the exudate is initially pale-yellow in colour, but as it solidifies, it becomes brown-black.

Jams. Herbal jams are solid or semi-solid preparations. The herbal paste or powder is cooked in liquid (water or milk), and ghee, sugar syrup, etc are added while cooking. A jam is ready when it achieves single or double thread consistency and when a dollop sinks into water *en masse* without spreading. A jam made of fresh ginger is a common household remedy used to strengthen the digestive fire, while another made of dry ginger powder is used as a winter tonic. There is a wide variety of jams used therapeutically for indigestion, diarrhoea, piles, bleeding disorders, respiratory problems, reproductive disorders, etc. *Chyavanaprasa*, the most well-known among jams, consists mainly of amla in addition to as many as forty herbs and at times, is fortified with even minerals. It is a rejuvenator and also a remedy for debility and old age.

Medicated Oils and Fats. Sneha are prepared by boiling a drug-fat-water mixture until the water evaporates and the remnants are strained. There are four textures distinguishable in Kerala preparations: flowing, soft, waxy and hard. While hair oils (often medicated with amla, Chinese rose, etc) are flowing, certain preparations like medicated ghee are in various semi-solid states (soft, waxy or hard). Soft fats are used for nasal medication. Waxy fats are used for internal consumption and the hard greasy ones are applied to the body. The hard fat often contains charred herbs.

Nasal and Eye Drops. Nasal and eye medication is preferred for purification in all diseases of the head, lungs, throat and eyes. A good daily routine includes introduction of a couple of drops of medicated oil or ghee into the nose or eyes as the case may be. Whenever any fresh juice is required to be introduced, sufficient caution is to be exercised to avoid any contamination. Sterilized cotton and clean hands are necessary. Never use more than 2–3 drops at a time.

Application of Warmed Leaves. Some leaves are applied on boils, etc after warming over a flame. The leaves which are otherwise hard or leathery get softened and pliable by such treatment and are rendered handy for bandaging the affected area. Sometimes a coating of oil (such as sesame oil) is applied on the surface of the leaves before warming them.

Burning the Plant Materials. This process is quite common and releases the aroma (e.g., resins, incense, etc) of the plant parts which helps in relieving nasal congestion, etc. In certain cases, plant parts are burnt over hot coals and the ash obtained is used as medicine.

Roasting the Plant Materials. Roasting plant parts such as seeds is a common method before they are used as medicine. By roasting in the skillet, the volatile oil content in seeds is gradually released and the efficacy of the plant parts, when used as medicine, increases. In Siddha medicine, roasting of leaves, etc is also done in mud pots. Such a roasting process removes traces of moisture, besides wilting the leaves.

A Note on Dosage

> *A doctor should treat taking account of the patient,*
> *the illness and the time.*
>
> —Tirukkural 949

Prescribing the optimal dosage of the plant material for a particular ailment and for the particular constitution of the patient has always been quite a challenging task for any herbalist. The main reason for this is the fact that the content of the so-called 'active principle' of a plant part varies widely due to factors such as climate, altitude, latitude, soil type, nutrition, temperature, relative humidity, season, time of plucking, packing, storage, etc. Determining the nature of the constitution of the patient has also been a crucial factor for determining the dosage of the drug.

As such, the dosage should vary from person to person and from drug to drug, the judgement being based on the close observation by the physician of the individual constitution and reaction of the patient, with a view to enhance or decrease the dose already prescribed by him. In other words, a close rapport between the physician and the patient is a *sine qua non* before making any such attempt. The practitioner should be fully aware of the inherent weakness in prescribing the dosage, or a particular dose of a drug, in a general or casual way, overlooking the importance of both the dynamism that a drug exhibits and the individuality of a patient's constitution. The crude manner in which dosage has been prescribed in this book is merely to broadly document roughly how much of the drug could be required. It has been assumed that the patient is fully grown and mature. The dosage indicated is therefore subject to modification by the prudent user.

Finally, I make no apologies for the fact that I approach patients like a 'primitive' shaman. For me, they represent highly complex psycho-physico-spiritual creatures rather than mechanical devices, taken up for servicing or repair. I am fully convinced that when a man suffers from an ailment, all he needs is relief best suited to his bodily constitution and in the least harmful way. It is in such a spirit that I hope readers too will approach the book.

Notes on Preparing Plant Parts

Collection. Although there are no hard and fast rules, the following principles are generally adhered to:

Roots, Rhizomes and Bark: They are collected in late autumn or early spring when vegetative growth has ceased.

Leaves and Flowering Tops: They are collected at the time of development of flowers and before maturing of fruit and seed as the photosynthetic activities are maximum at this time. The active principle content is also high.

Fruits: They are collected when fully grown, but unripe.

Seeds: They are collected when fully matured and if possible, before the fruits open for dispersal. Seed-like fruits such as coriander, saunf, ajwain, etc are harvested a little before they are fully ripe, to retain their fresh and bright appearance.

Drying: The object of drying is to remove moisture and to preserve the plant and its parts. Under natural conditions, the drug could be dried under the sun or in shade, according to the nature of its content or the active principle. Greater success is encountered in commercial drying, where the temperature and flow of air are controlled. Certain delicate drugs such as digitalis need a specific temperature for drying.

Garbling: The final stage in the processing of a drug is garbling. In this process, extraneous matter such as dirt, unwanted plant parts, adulterants, etc, are removed.

Packing: Different drugs need different types of packing. Basically, packing should ensure protection against moisture, fungus, insects, etc.

Storage and Preservation: Conditions for storage and preservation vary from plant to plant. In case of drugs such as digitalis, which deteriorate in the presence of moisture, the insertion of a suitable dehydrating substance in the container itself is a prerequisite. In general, the ideal conditions for preservation of all drugs are refrigeration or low temperatures.

Infusion: An infusion, like tea, is made by combining boiling water with herbs (usually the green parts or flowers) and steeping for 5 to 10 minutes to extract their active ingredients. Due to exposure to heat only for a short duration, this method ensures that the volatile elements and vitamins are not totally lost. It is recommended that a porcelain, enamel or glass pot be used while steeping the herbs. The pot should be covered with a tight-fitting lid to minimize evaporation. Sometimes sugar or honey can be added to the infusion to improve its taste. Most herb-teas (also called tisanes) are taken in small regular doses ranging from a teaspoon to a mouthful over a period of time. They are taken quite hot, if the intention is to break up a cold or cough. Otherwise they can be taken either lukewarm or cold.

Decoction: Hard materials such as wood-pieces, bark, roots, seeds, etc require prolonged boiling to extract their active ingredients. About $1/2$ cup of plant parts can be boiled in 1 cup water. It is better to use a non-metallic or enamelled pot. Green plant parts and flowers can be added to cold water, brought to a boil and allowed to remain so for 3–4 minutes. Or they can be added straight to boiling water and allowed to be immersed at a galloping boil for a few minutes. In either case the pot should be covered with a lid. Harder materials need to be boiled longer. Plant parts need to be strained out from the decoction. The Kerala physicians often strain the decoction and boil it again until it is reduced to one-and-a-half times the original weight of the herbs. For cooking decoctions clay pots are considered the best. However, copper pots for *kapha* problems, silver or bronze for *pitta* problems and gold or iron pot for *vata* problems are also considered acceptable and good.

Cold Extract: To ensure effective extraction of delicate or volatile compounds the herbs are steeped in a non-metallic or enamelled pot containing cold water (1:6 ratio of herb and water) for 8 to 12 hours. Strain and the drink is ready. Through this method, only minor amounts of mineral salts and bitter principles can be extracted. Compared to hot infusions, cold extracts would need double the quantity of plant material. This method is recommended for very delicate herbs such as hibiscus, sandalwood, jasmine, marigold, rose, coriander, vetiver, etc and for the treatment of *pitta* conditions.

Juice: While extracting juice from the plant material, a little cold water could be added. This is a good method for extracting water-soluble constituents, vitamins and minerals from the plant.

The juice should be consumed immediately after pressing, as otherwise the vitamin content is denatured and the fermentation process starts. This method is used in the case of all juicy plants particularly aloe, amlaki, brahmi, coriander, garlic, ginger, tulsi, lime, neem, onion, etc.

Syrup: The plant materials can be boiled in honey and strained through cheesecloth. This is an easier way of administering medicines to children.

Powder: Dried plant parts can be ground with the help of a traditional mortar and pestle or with a grinder or blender. Powders made from a combination of a number of drugs are popular in Ayurveda. The versatile *Triphala* is a shining example. The powder can be taken with water, milk or soup. It can be just swallowed with water or sprinkled on food. The common dosage is stated as the quantity that you can lift on the tip of a dinner-knife! These days, gelatine capsules can be used to facilitate swallowing. Sometimes powders are used externally as in the case of *Dashanga Lepa*, which contains liquorice, valerian, red sandalwood, cardamom, turmeric, etc. It is dusted on boils, mumps, abscesses, erysipelas and neuralgia.

Poultice: Also called cataplasm, the poultice is used to apply a herbal product to a skin area with moist heat. Often, the herb is made into a pulpy mass and warmed up. The warmed pulp is spread on a wet, hot cloth and wrapped around the affected area. In the case of mustard pulp or similar herbs, which are quite irritable to the skin, two layers of cloth could be used. After removing the poultice, the area could be washed with water or herbal tea to wipe out any left-over residue on the skin. Poultices are used to soothe, to irritate, or to draw out impurities from the body. Such an action depends on the type of herb selected for the purpose.

Fomentation: A Turkish towel can be soaked in a hot infusion or decoction and after wringing out the excess liquid, applied as hot as possible on the affected area.

Cold Compress: It is like fomentation, but the infusion or decoction used is cold. The cloth is left on the body until it is warmed by body heat. Usually it is left on for 10 to 15 minutes. This is repeated with another fresh cold compress.

Soap Substitutes. Certain plants contain a compound called saponin, which produces lather when the plant tissues are rubbed in water. They can also be used to make shampoos. The plants which contain saponin in sufficient quantity to produce lather are:

Papaya leaves

Soap-nut powder (reetha) and shikakai

Powder made of dried orange rind, lemon rind, rose petals, etc. All these can play an effective role as a substitute for soap.

Turmeric powder, which is a germicide, is also used along

with besan, *kasturi manjal*, etc. Powdered leaves of neem, curry-leaf, etc also find their use in substituting soap.

In combination with milk, these herbs make an ideal wash for the upkeep of skin and in preventing its damage due to weather, old age, bacteria, etc.

Volatile Oils: Volatile oils extracted from various plants have been in use from time immemorial. They are extracted by distilling grass (*Cymbopogon*, etc), leaves (basil, cinnamon, *Citrus*, etc), flowers (*Citrus*, jasmine, rose, saffron, etc), flower buds (lawsonia, mango, etc) fruits (black pepper, bel, cardamom, nutmeg, etc), seeds (anise, ajwain, coriander, cumin, saunf, etc), roots or rhizomes (galangal, ginger, sweet flag, turmeric, vetiver, etc), wood (agar, camphor, deodar, sandal, etc), bark (asafoetida, *boswellia*, camphor, commiphora, etc.)

The volatile oils are responsible for the characteristic odour of the plant. Some act on the Central Nervous System, increase appetite, aid digestion and regularize intestinal action. When placed on intact skin, they can increase the flow of blood, especially of leucocytes. This property associated with the bactericidal properties of certain oils is the basis of their antiseptic use.

Indian Acalypha

Acalypha indica

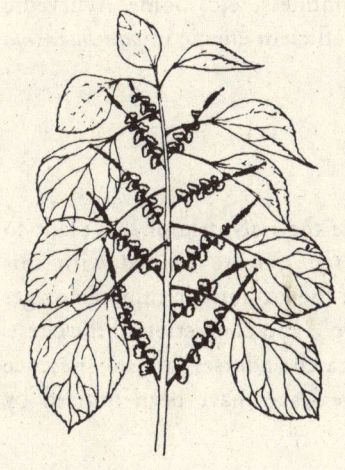

Harita manjari cures kapha.

—Svayamkriti

Cat-Sense?

Indian Acalypha is commonly called the Indian counterpart of catmint, a plant which cats are fond of. Due to their eating habits, cats often suffer from constipation and indigestion. It is curious indeed that whenever faced with such problems they search out this plant very much like a trained herbalist, uproot it and chew up the roots. The plant's Tamil name *Poonaivanangi* refers to its being 'worshipped' by the cat!

Drug from the Dunghill

Indian Acalypha is an unimpressive weed that grows on dunghills and manure-heaps. Its Tamil name *Kuppaimeni* refers to these unenviable habitats.

To the traditional village doctor, the Indian Acalypha is a handy drug. Both the leaves and roots of the plant are used for various purposes: to treat intestinal infections due to worms, to clean and disinfect the digestive tract, to fight phlegm, to initiate menstruation and to treat toothache, burns, stomach ache, hernia, *vata*-aggravation, asthma, bronchitis, pneumonia, rheumatism, itching, prurience, earache, numbness, etc. Some Ayurvedic practitioners use the leaves as an efficient emetic in *panchakarma* treatments.

Skin Cleanser

The tribes in the Nilgiri hills use the leaf-paste of this plant to clean their bodies. Their children too are washed with this leaf-paste. The women administer the leaf juice in minute dosages to children severely attacked by cold and congestion of the chest. It is interesting that scientific research endorses this: the presence of antibacterial principles in the leaves have been noticed by bacteriologists.

Profile

Botanical Name	:	*Acalypha indica* Linn.	
English Name	:	Indian Acalypha.	
Indian Names	:	Bengali	: *Muktabarsi, Muktajhuri*
		Gujarati	: *Vanchi Kanto*
		Hindi	: *Khokali, Kuppi*
		Kannada	: *Kuppi, Kuppigida*
		Malayalam	: *Kuppameni*
		Marathi	: *Khokhali*
		Oriya	: *Indramaris*

Sanskrit	:	*Harita Manjari*
Tamil	:	*Arimanjari, Kuppaimeni, Kuppaveni, Meni, Poonaivanangi*
Telugu	:	*Kuppichettu, Kuppinta, Kuppintaku, Muripindi.*

Family	:	Euphorbiaceae.
Appearance	:	Annual weed, reaching a height of about 60 cm. Leaves, deep green in colour, oval to round in shape, serrated at the edges and arranged in a beautiful rosette. Flowers, green and inconspicuous, arranged on a long stalk. The plant has a spreading root system which does not penetrate deep into the soil, enabling even a kitten to pull it out easily. Seeds aplenty, scattered on the ground, awaiting showers.
Distribution	:	Found in the plains and in peninsular India, the plant is known as a weed in farmlands and gardens. Also found by roadsides and in wastelands.
Medicinal Parts	:	The whole plant, collected at the time of flowering, especially the leaves and roots.

In Tradition

AILMENT	PRESCRIPTION
❧ Bed sores	: Dust a fine powder of the dried leaves on the affected areas frequently.
❧ Bleeding piles	: Boil 1 cup each of the juices of Indian Acalypha, tulsi leaves and castor oil till the mixture achieves the consistency of

3

honey. Cool and bottle. *Dose:* 2 tsp along with 1 cup hot milk at bedtime for 5 days.

❧ Boils, inflammation in legs, insect bite : Grind the leaves into a fine paste. Add a little slaked lime and apply locally.

❧ Constipation, intestinal worms, phlegm : Soak a few leaves in drinking water for a couple of hours. Take 1 to 2 tsp of the infusion. (*Caution:* In excess, this may cause vomiting. Please note that the plant has a laxative effect.)

❧ Eczema, psoriasis, ringworm, skin diseases : Grind some leaves and 1 tsp salt into a fine paste and apply on the affected parts.

❧ Headache : Express the leaf juice and apply on the affected areas.

❧ Intestinal worms : Dry the leaves and make into a fine powder. Take $1/4$ to $1/2$ tsp with lukewarm water. (*Caution:* It has a purgative action.)

❧ Intestinal worms, stomach infections : Grind a few leaves along with a few garlic pods and eat with cooked rice. (*Caution:* It may work as a purgative.)

❧ Muscular pain : Extract the juice from the leaves and mix with an equal quantity of gingelly oil. Boil the mixture till the moisture evaporates. Apply on the affected parts while bearably hot.

❧ Phlegm : Mix the leaf juice with a little neem oil. Dip a cotton-bud into it and apply carefully over the throat/root of the tongue before retiring.

❧ Piles : Grind equal quantities of the dried leaves of Indian Acalypha and tulsi into a very fine powder. Take 2 or 3 pinches with a little ghee thrice daily for a few days. (*Note:* During this treatment please avoid intoxicants like coffee, tea, cigarettes, alcohol, etc. and ensure proper sleep at night.)

❧ Rashes : Make a poultice of fresh leaves and apply on the affected parts.

❧ Rashes, skin-eruptions : Mix equal quantities of the juices of Indian Acalypha and tulsi with the same quantity of castor oil. Boil the mixture thoroughly till the moisture has evaporated. Apply this oil on the affected parts. Simultaneously, 1/4 tsp of this oil can also be administered orally with 1 cup cow's milk.

❧ Tinea versicolor : Grind equal parts of Acalypha leaves and common salt into a fine paste and apply on the affected areas.

❧ *Vata*-aggravation : Press a few leaves along with salt and extract the juice. Instil 1 or 2 drops in both nostrils every morning for a few days.

❧ Venereal sores : Grind the leaves into a fine paste and apply locally.

♣ Wounds, itching   : Grind the leaves with turmeric into a fine paste and apply.

Note. Individual results may vary.

A Word of Caution

The leaves can cause severe vomiting and purgation in excess.

In Science

Central Council for Research in Indian Medicine and Homoeopathy. 1978. *Tribal Pockets of Nilgiris—Recordings of the Field Study on Medicinal Flora and Health Practices.* New Delhi. (Ethno-botany.)

Chopra, R. N. et al. 1956. *Glossary of Indian Medicinal Plants.* New Delhi: CSIR. (Laxative, expectorant properties studied.)

George, M. et al. 1947. Investigations of Plant Antibiotics (Part II). A search for antibiotic substances in some Indian medicinal plants. *J. Sci. Industr. Res.* 6B(3):42–46. (Leaf extracts fight the bacteria: *S. aureus* and *E. coli.*)

John, D. 1984. One hundred useful raw drugs of the Kani tribes of Trivandrum forest division. *Int. J. Crude Drug Res.* 22(1):17–39. (Medicated oil containing the leaf juice cures skin diseases.)

Masilamani, G. et al. 1981. Study of *Karapan* (eczema). *J. Res. Ayur. Siddha* 2(2):109–121. (Leaf juice expressed with a little common salt is found useful in eczema.)

Nateswar, K. et al. 1982. Preliminary studies on the action of *Acalypha indica*—A folklore drug. *Nagarjun* 26(3):62–63. (The use of the drug as a cardiac stimulant.)

Raman, K. G. et al. 1979. A pilot study of *Kuppaimeni* (*Acalypha indica*) in *Swasakasam* (Bronchial asthma). *J. Res. Indian Med. Yoga and*

Homoeo. 14(3–4):81–86. (Decoction of the green leaves relieves wheezing cough.)

Rao, Y. M. and D. R. Krishna. 1979. Study of the antibacterial activity of the extract of the plant *Acalypha indica. J. Sci. Res. Pl. and Med.* 3(2&3):51–53. (Eliminates pathogens.)

Ravishankar, V. 1982. Hypertension and its treatment—a review from Siddha texts. *Nagarjun* 26(3):57–61. (Blood pressure brought down.)

Sairam, T. V. 1998. Indian Acalypha. *Dignity Dialogue*, July 14–15.

2

Chirchita
Achyranthes aspera

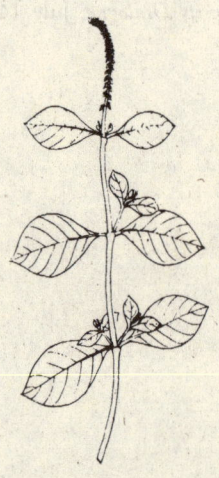

Brushing the teeth with young
branchlets of apamargah will
benefit one and all.

—Kurma Purana 18.20.
(6th Century A.D.)

The Ugly Duckling

To the uninitiated, a chirchita plant may appear like the proverbial
ugly duckling, with minute hairs all over its shoot system. It
may also irritate passersby with its barbed prickles which hook
themselves effortlessly onto one's clothes. In due recognition of
these features, Sanskrit has several names for this plant:
apamargah, the one that hinders pedestrians; *pratyakaparni*, the
one with leaves at right angles to the stem; *kisaparni*, the one
hairy as a monkey and *mayurakah*, the one whose floral stock
resembles the head of a peacock.

Chirchita is quite popular in indigenous medicine, particularly with the Kotas of the Nilgiri Hills, who value the entire plant for its medicinal properties.

The Santhals of Madhya Pradesh use the plant in the treatment of snakebite. The plant is also reportedly used by them to treat blindness in cattle (Jain and Tarafder, 1970).

The Khasi and Garo of Meghalaya use the plant for curing several skin-afflictions including the dreadful leprosy (Rao, 1981).

In Orissa, tribal women who wish to prevent pregnancy use the juice extracted from the root (Prem Kishore et al. 1982). In Bastar, the whole root is inserted into the vagina to induce abortion (Jain, 1965).

From the Jungle to the Lab

Several clinical investigations conducted on chirchita in modern research laboratories in several parts of the world—Africa, China, India, Philippines, etc. have upheld autochthonous wisdom in employing this plant as a medicine. Experiments have also revealed that achyranthine, an alkaloid extracted from this plant, can help lower blood pressure and heart-rate, by dilating the blood vessels and increasing the rate of respiration.

Profile

Botanical Names	:	*Achyranthes aspera* Linn.
		Achyranthes bidenta Bl.
English Name	:	Prickly Chaff-Flower Plant.
Indian Names	:	Hindi : *Chirchita, Chichinda*
		Kannada : *Uttarani*
		Malayalam : *Katalati, Valiyakatalati, Venkatalati*

9

Sanskrit	:	*Apamargah*
Tamil	:	*Naayuruvi*
Telugu	:	*Apamarga.*
Family	:	Amaranthaceae.
Appearance	:	Erect hairy herb; leaves, opposite, covered with soft hairs. Flowers, small, greenish-white. Fruit, egg-like.
Distribution	:	Found almost everywhere in the wastelands, especially in the plains.
Medicinal Parts	:	Whole plant, root and seeds.
Ayurvedic Preparations	:	*Ardhavilvam Kashayam, Aaviltolaadi Bhasmam, Jaatyaadi Tailam, Surasaadi Tailam, Svarnamuktaadi Gulika.*

In Tradition

AILMENT	PRESCRIPTION
❧ Bleeding piles	: Grind the leaves into a fine paste. Mix some gingelly oil into the paste. Apply on the affected areas twice a day for 7 days.
❧ Cholera	: Mix 1 tsp finely powdered root in warm water and drink.
❧ Cholera, stomach disorders, urine retention	: Clean the root and grind it into a fine paste. Stir 1 tsp into a glass of lukewarm water. Allow it to infuse for 10 minutes and drink the clear liquid. Twice daily.
❧ Cold, cough, fever	: Make an infusion of 1 tbsp leaves/flowers in 1 cup water and drink.

❧ Cough

: Mix 1 tsp root powder along with $1/4$ tsp black pepper and 1 tsp honey. Take twice or thrice a day.

: Burn the root. Mix $1/2$ tsp of the ash with 1 tsp honey and take twice or thrice a day.

❧ Deafness of certain types, ear infection

: Burn the plant and mix 2 tsp of the ash along with 2 tbsp gingelly oil and heat. Cool, strain, and use as ear drops. (*Caution:* Take the necessary precautions to prevent infection.)

❧ Diarrohea and dysentry (early stages)

: Take the powdered leaves (1 tsp). Mix with 1 tsp honey. Take twice or thrice a day.

❧ Dropsy

: Boil 4 tbsp of the whole plant in 1 teacup water for 20 to 30 minutes. Take the strained liquid (about 2 tbsp) twice a day.

❧ Fever

: Grind the fresh leaves into a fine paste. Take 1 tsp of the paste with 2 tsp powdered jaggery.

❧ Insect bite, scorpion sting, psoriasis

: Grind the leaves into a fine paste and apply on the affected parts.

❧ Nosebleeds

: Burn the plant and mix 2 tsp ash into 2 tbsp gingelly oil and heat well. Cool, strain and use as nasal drops. (*Caution:* Take the necessary precautions to prevent infection.)

11

❦ Partial paralysis   : Grind the root in fine powder. Mix $1/4$ tsp of this with 1 black peppercorn (finely powdered) and 1 tsp milk. Use as nasal drops.
(*Note:* Proper physiotherapy may also be necessary.)

❦ Piles   : Mix 1 tsp crushed seeds into your normal food and eat.

         : Stir 1 tsp crushed seeds into 1 glass of the water used for washing rice, and drink.

         : Burn the roots to obtain the ash. Apply on the affected areas.

❦ Spleen enlargement : Grind the dried plant into a fine powder. Mix 2 tbsp of this powder with a little beaten curd or buttermilk and take twice daily for a few days.

❦ Stomach ache   : Take 2 tbsp fresh leaf juice. Dilute it with water (1:4) and drink every day.

❦ Toothache   : Crush the end of a piece of fresh root and chew frequently.

❦ Wounds   : Clean the wounds with the leaf juice. Then bandage with leaves.

Note: Individual results may vary.

A Word of Caution

Pregnant women are advised to avoid the use of chirchita.

In Science

Aminuddin, R. D. G. and S. A. Khan. 1992. Ethno-medicinal uses of *Achyranthes aspera* L. in Orissa (India). *Intl. J. Pharmocognosy* 30(2):113–115. (Ethno-medicinal documentation.)

Anon. 1975. *Herbal Pharmacy in the People's Republic of China*. U.S.A.: National Academy of Sciences.

Asim, F. et al. 1983. Anti-microbial activity of certain Sudanese plants used in folkloric medicine, screening for antibacterial activity (1). *Filoterapia* 54(1):3–7. (The plant's role in inhibiting the spread of bacteria.)

Basu, N. K. et al. 1957. Chemical investigation of *Achyranthes aspera*. *J. Proc. Inst. Chemistry* (India) 29:55–58.

Bhide, N. K. et al. 1976. Quoted from *Medicinal Plants of India*. I, 12. New Delhi: Indian Council of Medical Research. (Facilitates urine outflow.)

Central Council for Research in Ayurveda and Siddha. 1996. *Pharmacological Investigations of Certain Medicinal Plants & Compound Formulations used in Ayurveda and Siddha*. New Delhi. (Medicinal evaluation of the plant.)

Central Council for Research in Indian Medicine and Homoeopathy. 1978. *Tribal Pockets of Nilgiris—Recordings of the Field Study on Medicinal Flora and Health Practices*. New Delhi. (Documents widespread use among the Nilgiri hill people.)

Chagnon, M. 1984. Pharmacological screening of medicinal plants of Rwanda. *J. Ethno-Pharmacol.* 12(3):239–251. (Useful in controlling colic.)

Chakraborty, H. L. 1975. Herbal Heritage of India. *Bull. Bot. Soc. Bengal* 29(1):97–103.

Chatterjee, B. N. 1980. Role of cystone in various urinary disorders. *Probe* 22(1) 27–30. (Cystone, an Ayurvedic preparation containing chirchita, is clinically found to completely cure urolithiasis, crystalluria and urinary tract infections.)

Chopra, R. N. et al. 1969. *Glossary of Indian Medicinal Plants*. New Delhi: Council of Scientific and Industrial Research. Supplement 2. (Fights colic and bronchial infections.)

Dhar, M. L. et al. 1968. Screening of Indian plants for biological activity. Part I. *Indian J. Exptl. Biol.* 6:232. (Reduces the sugar-level of diabetics.)

Gambhir, S. S. et al. 1965. Pharmacological study of *Achyranthes aspera* Linn.—A Preliminary Report. *Indian J. Physiol. Pharmacol.* 9:185. (Eases urine outflow.)

Gopalachari, R. and M. L. Dhar. 1958. Studies on the constitution of the saponin from the seeds of *Achyranthes aspera*: Part I—Identification of the sapogenin. *J. Sci. Industr. Res.* 17B:276–278.

———. 1952. Chemical examination of the seeds of *Achyranthes aspera* Linn. *J. Sci. Industr. Res.* 11B:209.

———. 1952. Chemical examination of *Achyranthes aspera*. *J. Sci. Industr. Res.* 11B:209.

Gupta, S. S. and I. Khanijo. 1970. Antagonistic effect of *Achyranthes aspera* on intestinal contractility induced by oxytocin. *Indian J. Physiol. Pharmacol.* 14:63.

Gupta, S. S. et al. 1972. Diuretic effect of saponin of *Achyranthes aspera* (*Apamarga*). *Indian J. Pharmac.* 4:208. (Facilitates the excretion of sodium and potassium in urine.)

———. 1972. Cardiac stimulant activity of the saponin of *Achyranthes aspera* Linn. *Indian J. Med. Res.* 60:462. (The hypotensive activity of the plant recorded.)

Herrera, C. L. et al. 1984. Philippine plants as possible sources of anti-fertility agents. *Philipp. J. Sci.* 113(1–2):91–129. (Prevents urine blockage.)

Ikram, M. and I. Haq. 1980. Screening of medicinal plants for anti-microbial activity. Part I. *Filoterapia* 51(5):276–278. (Stops the growth of the bacteria: *S. dysenteriae*, *B. subtilis*, *E. coli* and *S. typhi*.)

Jain, S. K. 1965. Medicinal plantlore of the tribals of Bastar. *Econ. Bot.* 19(3):236–250. (How the plant helps check unwanted conception.)

Jain, S. K. and C. R. Tarafder. 1970. Medicinal plantlore of the Santhals. *Econ. Bot.* 24(3):241–278. (A cure for tiger-bite and snakebite.)

Kapil, V. B. et al. 1976. Some important aromatic and medicinal plants of the Kumaon hills and its surroundings. *Indian Perfum.* 20 (Part 2):1–7. (Bactericidal properties highlighted.)

Khastgir, H. N. et al. 1958. Sapogenin from seeds of *Achyranthes aspera*. *J. Indian Chem.* Soc. 35:693–694.

Manandhar, N. P. 1993. Herbal remedies of Surkhet District, Nepal. *Filoterapia* 64(3):276–278.

Misra, T. N. et al. 1990. Antifungal essential oil and long-chain alcohol from *Achyranthes aspera*. *Phytochemistry* 31(5):1811–1812. (The plant's role in fighting fungus.)

Ojha, D. and G. Singh. 1968. *Apamarga (Achyranthes aspera)* in the treatment of Lepromatous Leprosy. *Lep. Rev.* 39:23. (Decoction of the whole plant tested on 36 leprosy patients showed encouraging results in all cases.)

Ojha, D. et al. 1966. Role of an indigenous drug (*Achyranthes aspera*) in the management of reactions of leprosy—Preliminary Observations. *Lep. Rev.* 37:115. (An innocuous, roadside herb can fight leprosy effectively.)

Oliver-Bever, B. 1983. Medicinal plants of tropical West Africa, II. Plants acting on the nervous system. *J. Ethno Pharmacol.* 7(1):1–93 (The efficacy of the seeds.)

Oommachan, M. and S. S. Khan. 1981. Plants in aid of family planning. *Ancient Sci. Life.* I(1):64–66.

Pakrashi, A. and N. Bhattacharya. 1977. Abortifacient principle of *Achyranthes aspera* Linn. *Indian J. Exp. Biol.* 15:856. (A seminal contribution.)

Prakash, A. O. 1986. Potentialities of some indigenous plants for anti-fertility activity. *Int. J. Crude Drug Res.* 24(1):19–24. (Prevented the development of pregnancy in 60% of the experimental animals.)

Prasad, S. and I. C. Bhattacharya. 1959. Pharmacognostic study of *Achyranthes aspera. Indian J. Pharm.* 21(3):85.

Prem Kishore. et al. 1982. Oral contraceptive folk claims from Puri district. Orissa. *Bull. Medico-Ethno Bot. Res.* 3(1):65–67. (The juice of the root is an effective abortifacient.)

Rao, R. R. 1981. Ethno-botany of Meghalaya: medicinal plants used by the Khasi and Garo tribes. *Econ. Bot.* 35(1):4–9. (The root powder when mixed with crushed snails and applied locally is reported to cure leprosy.)

Sairam, T. V. 1997. Apmargah-Achyranthes aspera L. *Mystic India*, Oct. 81–83.

Sairam, T. V. 1998. Apmargah. *Dignity Dialogue*, April 15–16.

Satyavati, G. V. 1984. Indian plants and plant products with anti-fertility effect. *Ancient Sci. Life* 3(4):276–278. (The plant can be used to slow down the rate of population growth.)

Singh, K. K. and S. C. Singh. 1980. Some medicinal plants in the folklore of Varanasi District U.P. *Bull. Medico Ethno Bot. Res.* 91:28–34. (How unwanted pregnancies are prevented.)

Thakur, R. S. et al. 1989. *Major Medicinal Plants of India*. Lucknow: C.I.M.A.P.

Tripathi, R. M. et al. 1970. Effect of saponin of *Achyranthes aspera* (*Apamarga*) against adrenalin-induced anti-diuresis in rats. *Assoc. Physiol. and Pharmacol. (India)*:15.

Wadhwa, V. et al. 1986. Contraceptive and hormonal properties of *Achyranthes aspera* in rats and hamsters. *Planta Med:* 3:231–233. (A herbal contraceptive.)

Wilson, R. T. and W. G. Mariam. 1979. Medicine and magic in central Tigre—A contribution to the ethno-botany of the Ethiopian plateau. *Econ. Bot.* 33(1):29–34.

3

Calamus

Acorus calamus

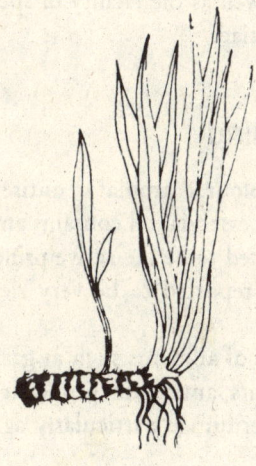

Vacha, the memory-enhancer.

—Raja Vallabham

Roots and Traditions

The roots of calamus lead back to Europe. Yet it has so admirably merged into the ancient medical systems in India and China that its popularity as a folk medicine has always stood very high in these parts of the globe as well.

The officinal part of the drug is the rootstock, which finds mention in the medical literatures of China and India.

Sanskrit names the plant after its various qualities: 'auspicious', 'born from water', 'destroyer of spirits', 'harsh', 'intense odour', 'intellect-awakener', 'success'—just to mention a few!

The drug successfully reduces *vata* and *kapha* but increases *pitta*. It is recommended by vaids for the improvement of memory-power and the functioning of the brain and nervous system. The powder is blown into the nose to help a patient in shock or coma regain consciousness. The drug fights against toxins accumulated in the body over a period of time. It works effectively against cough and pyorrhoea. Dreaded diseases like elephantiasis, hepatitis, etc. are also treated with this drug. It improves the timbre of the voice as well as the faculty of speech. It is also believed to be an aphrodisiac.

Medicine for Body and Mind

The dry rootstock yields a yellow-coloured aromatic, antiseptic, volatile oil on steam distillation. The essential oil contains among other things, asarone, which is reported to be the active principle of the plant. Indian calamus oil is reported to be very rich in asarone, with as much as 82%.

The oil is effective against a host of ailments such as gastritis and various skin diseases due to its antiseptic properties. It promotes digestion. It works as a vermifuge particularly against bedbugs, moths and lice.

Calamus oil is an acknowledged nerve-stimulant, helpful in mental concentration exercises. The drug is believed to ward off evil spirits (*bhutas*) and to cure hysteria and insanity due to its powerful impact on the brain and nervous system.

Medicine for Babies

In Tamil, calamus is referred to as *pillai-marundu*, medicine for infants. To prepare this formulation, the experienced vaidyar paints a smooth coat of castor oil all over the rootstock. He then chars it over a flame. The resultant ash is the drug which is known as *ukkiram*. A paste made by mixing this powder with ghee is normally administered to infants in the villages as the first post-natal ritual. This paste is believed to sharpen the intellect of the infant.

Profile

Botanical Name	:	*Acorus calamus* L.
English Names	:	Sweet-Flag, Sweet-Rush, Calamus.
Indian Names	:	Assamese : *Themeprii*
		Bengali : *Bach*
		Gujarati : *Gandhilovaj, Godavaj*
		Hindi : *Gorbach, Safedbach, Vacha*
		Kannada : *Baje, Bajegida, Baji*
		Kashmiri : *Vabi*
		Malayalam : *Vayampu, Vashampu*
		Marathi &
		Punjabi : *Bariboj, Vach, Vekhand*
		Urdu : *Bacha*
		Sanskrit : *Ugragandha, Vacha*
		Tamil : *Vasambu*
		Telugu : *Basa, Vadaja, Vasa.*
Family	:	Araceae.
Appearance	:	A marshy, fragrant herb. Leaves, simple, alternate, linear, glossy bright green. Flowers, fragrant, pale green on a stump. Fruit, a 3-celled fleshy capsule. Rootstock, pinkish brown, white and spongy inside.
Distribution	:	Commonly found in Kashmir, Karnataka and Manipur.
Medicinal Part	:	Rootstock.

19

In Tradition

AILMENT	PRESCRIPTION
↓ Blood impurities	: Apply a thick coat of turmeric paste on a piece of calamus root. Dry in the sun and then roast over a flame till charred. Remove from the fire and grind into a very fine powder. Bottle and take 3–4 pinches twice a day for 21 days.
↓ Bronchitis, headache, pneumonia, rheumatic joints	: Apply a paste of calamus root on the affected areas.
↓ Cholera	: Crush 1 tsp root and boil with 4 glasses of water. Strain and drink 1/4 glass every 15 minutes 3 or 4 times.
↓ Colic, flatulence, stomach upset	: Burn a piece of the root till charred. Mix with a little castor (or coconut) oil and apply over the lower abdomen.
↓ Cough, fever, stomach ache	: Boil 1/4 tsp each of the powders of the roots of calamus and liquorice in 2 glasses of water. Cool and sip 4 tbsp two to three times a day. (*Note:* 1 tsp honey can be added.)
↓ Cough in children	: Mix 2 pinches of *ukkiram* with an equal quantity of honey and administer in 3 doses a day.
↓ Cough, throat irritation	: Lick a small piece of the root. (*Note:* This activates salivary functioning.)

❦ Diarrhoea,
fever, gas,
indigestion,
speech-defects

: Take 2–3 pinches of the root powder
with honey every morning on an empty
stomach.

❦ Dysentery,
indigestion,
noise in the
stomach,
rheumatism

: Powder equal quantities of calamus
root, pippali, black pepper, dried
ginger, rind of chebulic myrobalan and
rock-salt and store. Take $1/4$ tsp of this
mixture with 1 teacup warm water or
1 tsp honey.

❦ Ear infection,
pus in ears

: Grind equal quantities of the roots of
the drumstick tree, calamus and garlic
and warm in some gingelly oil. When
bearably warm, drench in cotton and
use as ear drops.

❦ Gas, intestinal
worms, nervous
weakness

: Take 1–2 pinches of ukkiram with
some hot water.

❦ Gas problems

: Mix 2 pinches of *ukkiram* and 1 tsp
dried ginger powder. Add some sugar.
Take with a little water.

❦ Hair loss

: Mix 1 tsp powdered root in 2 tbsp cold
coconut milk and make a paste. Apply
on the affected parts and allow it to
remain for $1/2$ hour before rinsing it off.

❦ Indigestion, loss
of appetite,
stomach upset

: Mix $1/2$ tsp powdered root in 1 litre
cold water, raise to the boil and allow
to stand. Drink a cup 3–4 times.

❦ Indigestion,
stomach upset

Burn and char the root powder. *Dose:*
1–2 pinches with honey or hot water.

21

❧ Nervous weakness : Take 1–2 pinches of the powdered root with a little water twice a day for 40 days.

❧ Risk of infections : Lick at a small piece of the root. (*Note:* As a prophylactic.)

❧ Syphilis : Grind equal quantities of ashwagandha, calamus and kustha into a fine powder. Mix in some butter (obtained from buffalo-milk) to make a smooth paste. Apply this ointment over the affected parts.

❧ Ulcers, wounds : Dust a fine powder of the root over the affected areas.

Note: Individual results may vary.

A Word of Caution

Certain active agents of the plant are feared to be carcinogenic. Use of this drug without consulting a qualified physician may prove harmful.

Even in small doses (say 30 grains) the drug can induce emesis.

In Science

Agarwal, S. L. et al. 1956. Preliminary studies of certain pharmacological actions of *Acorus calamus*. *J American Pharm. Assn.* 45:655–656.

Arora, R. C. et al. 1986. *Acorus calamus*—a lipid lowering agent. *J. Res. Edn. Ind. Med.* 5(2):33–35. (Calamus fights cholesterol.)

Athanossova-Shopova, S. and K. Roussinov. 1965. Pharmacological studies on Bulgarian plants with a view to their anticonvulsant effect. *Compt. Rand. Acad. Bulg. Sci.* 18(7):691–694; *Biol. Abstr.* 48(1):2517. 1967. (The uses of Bulgarian calamus.)

Bauxter, R. M. et al. 1960. Separation of hypnotic potentiating principle from the essential oil of *Acorus calamus* Linn. of Indian origin by liquid-gas chromatography. *Nature* 185:466. (Chemistry of the oil.)

Bhattacharya, I. C. 1968. Effect of *Vacha* (Acorus) oil on the amphetamine induced agitation, hexo-barbital sleeping time and instrumental avoidance conditioning in rats. *J. Res. Indian Med.* 2(2):195–202. (Protective action.)

Bose, B. C. et al. 1960. Some aspects of chemical and pharmacological studies of *Acorus calamus* Linn. *J. Amer. Pharm. Ass. Sci. Ed.* 49:32–34. (Its use as a muscle-relaxant.)

Boyuan, Hu Ji Yaoyuan. 1986. A research on anti-carcinogenic activation of *Acorus calamus* of alpha asarone on human carcinoma cells. *Chin. J. Integ. Trad. West. Med.* 6(8):480–483. (Anti-cancer.)

Chak, I. M. and J. N. Sharma. 1965. Effect of asarone on experimentally induced conflict neurosin in rats. *Indian J. Exp. Biol.* 3:252. (Tranquillizing effect on rats.)

Chopra, I. C. et al. 1957. Antibacterial properties of volatile principles from *Alpinia galanga* and *Acorus calamus*. *Antibiotics Chemotherapy* 7:378. (Uproots harmful bacteria.)

————. 1954. Pharmacological action of some common essential oil-bearing plants used in indigenous medicine. *Indian J. Med. Res.* 42:381.

Chopra, R. N. et al. 1956. *Glossary of Indian Medicinal Plants*. New Delhi: CSIR. 5. (Use of calamus in snakebite; as an insecticide particularly in the case of bedbugs, moths and lice; as a sedative, analgesic, and anticonvulsant.)

Dandiya, P. C. et al. 1958. Studies in *Acorus calamus* I. Phytochemical investigations. *Can. J.Pharm.* 91:607. (The nature of calamus oil.)

————. 1959. Studies on *Acorus calamus*. Part II. Investigation of volatile oil. *J. Pharm. (London)* 11(3):163–168. (Action on the Central Nervous System.)

Dandiya, P. C. and J. D. Sharma. 1962. Studies on *Acorus calamus.* V. Pharmacological actions of asarone and Beta-asarone on central nervous system. *Indian J. Med. Res.* 50(1):46–60. (No analgesic action observed by the researchers.)

Dandiya, P. C. and M. K. Menon. 1964. Actions of asarone on behaviour, stress and hyperthermia and its interaction with central stimulants. *J. Pharmacol. Exptl. Therap.* 145:42. (The effect of asarone on mind and behaviour.)

————. 1964. Some more pharmacological action of asarone, the active principle of *Acorus calamus. Indian J. Physiol. and Pharmacol.* 8:44. (Properties as a sedative.)

————. 1965. Interaction of asarone with mescaline, amphetamine and themorine. *Life Sci.* 4:1635. (Properties as a sedative.)

Das, P. K. et al. 1962. Spasmolytic activity of asarone and essential oil of *Acorus calamus* Linn. *Arch. Int. Pharmacodyn.* 135:167. (As a cardiac depressant.)

Das Gupta, S. R. 1977. Preliminary studies of the effect of a chloroform-extracted factor from *Acorus calamus* on the behaviour of conscious rhesus monkeys. *Sci. and Cult.* 43(5):218–219.

Das Gupta, S. R. and B. B. Patra. 1975. Studies on the pharmacological action on the chloroform-extracted factor of *Acorus calamus* on cardiovascular system. *62nd session of the Indian Sci. Congress Association.* (Beneficial action on the cardiovascular system.)

Dey, D. and M. N. Das. 1980. Pharmacognostic studies of *Acorus calamus.* Calcutta: *Proc. 67th Session. Indian Sci. Congress.* (As a powerful drug.)

Dhalla, N. S. and I. S. Bhattacharya. 1968. Further studies on neuro-pharmacological actions of Acorus oil. *Arch. Int. Pharmacodyn.* 172:356. (As a tranquillizer.)

Dighe, P. Y. et al. 1955. Fungistatic properties of Acorus calamus. *Bull. Nat. Inst. Sci. India 4.*

Dombek, C. and L. Liberti. 1990. Calamus. *Lawrence Review of Nat. Prod.* 1–2.

Gupta, J. C. et al. 1955. Essential oil from the rhizomes of *Acorus calamus. J. Proc. Oil Technol. Assn.* 11:31–33.

Iguchi, M. et al. 1969. Isolation and structure of iso-calamendiol. *Tetrahedron Lett.* 3729. (Composition of the oil.)

Jain, S. R. et al. 1974. Antibacterial evaluation of some indigenous volatile oils. *Planta Med.* 26(2):196–199. (Fights several harmful bacteria: *P. solanaceum, C. diphtheriae, S. typhi and S. albus.*)

Joshi, C. G. and N. G. Nagar. 1952. Antibiotic activity of some Indian medicinal plants. *J. Sci. Industr. Res.* 11b(6):261. (Fights *Staphylococcus aureus.*)

Khare, A. K. et al. 1982. Experimental evaluation of antiepileptic activity of Acorus oil. *J. Sci. Res. Plant Med.* 3(4):100–103. (Fights epilepsy.)

Kiuchi, F. et al. 1991. Screening of crude drugs used in Nepal for nematocidal activity on the larva of *Toxocara canis. Shoyakugaku Zasshi* 43(4):294–299. (Kills worms.)

Madan, B. R. et al. 1960. Anticonvulsant, antiveratrinic and antiarrhythmic action of *Acorus calamus* Linn., an indigenous drug. *Arch. Int. Pharmacodyn.* 124(1–2):201–211; *Biol. Abstr.* 35(10):4666,1960. (Action on the Central Nervous System.)

Mamgain, P. and R. H. Singh, 1994. Controlled clinical trial of the *Lekhaniya Drug Vaca (Acorus calamus)* in cases of ischaemic heart-diseases. *J. Res. Ayur. Sid.* XV. 1&2:35–51. (In the management of ischaemic heart-diseases.)

Menon, M. K. and P. C. Dandiya. 1963. Tranquillizing properties of asarone and beta-asarone, active constituents of *Acorus calamus. Indian J. Physiol. Pharmacol.* 7:14. (Tranquillizer in calamus.)

———. 1967. The mechanism of the tranquillizing action of asarone from *Acorus calamus* Linn. *J. Pharm. Pharmacol.* 9:170. (How calamus affects the Central Nervous System.)

———. 1965. Studies of Acorus calamus-Mechanism of the tranquillizing action of asarone. *Indian J. Physiol. Pharmac.* 10(2):7.

Minato, H. et al. 1971. Components of the root of *Acorus calamus.* *Chem Pharm. Bull.* 19:638. (Column chromatography on alumina yields new compounds.)

Mukherjee, T. D. and Govind Ram. 1960. Studies on indigenous insecticidal plants Part III. *Acorus calamus* Linn. *J. Sci. Industr. Res.* 19C:112. (Bedbugs, moths and lice are killed by calamus.)

Nadkarni, A. K. 1954. *Indian Materia Medica.* Bombay.

Patra, B. B. et al. 1975. Observation of a new flavanoid compound from *Acorus calamus* on behaviour of conscious animals. *VIII Annual Conference of Indian Pharmacological Society.* 1975.

————. 1976. Studies on the pharmacological action of chloroform extracted factor of *Acorus calamus* on smooth muscles. *Proc. of the Indian Sci. Congress Assoc.* (Relaxes muscles.)

————. 1979. Some observations on the pharmacological activity of a flavone from *Acorus calamus.* New Delhi: XI Annual Conf. of Indian Pharmacol. Soc. 1978. *Indian J. Pharmacol.* 11:51. (Tranquillizer-like activity.)

————. 1979. Neuropharmacological studies with a flavone of *Acorus calamus.* Institute of Med. Sci. BHU: *Seminar on Drug Potentials of Indian Medicinal Plants.* (Favours from flavone.)

Pivenko, G. P. et al. 1957. The chemical and antibacterial properties of the essential oil of Acorus root. *Trudy Kharkov. Farmatsevt. Inst. No.* I:294–299. *Chem. Abstr.* 53:4425a. 1959. (The oil kills the Streptococcal spore and the Tubercle bacillus.)

Prakash, C. 1981. A note on preliminary study on *Acorus calamus* L in the treatment of bronchial asthma. *J. Res. Ayur. Siddha* 1(2):329–330 (Fights asthma.)

Raquibuddoula, M. et al. 1967. Solvent extraction of oil of *Acorus calamus.* *J. Sci. Res. Dacca (Pakistan)* 4:234. (Oil-chemistry.)

Roy, A. K. and S. K. Chourasia. 1990. Mycotoxin incidence in root drugs. *Intl. J. Crude Drug Res.* 28(2):157–160.

Sairam, T. V. 1997. Acorus Calamus. *Dignity Dialogue.*

Saxena, B. P. et al. 1977. A new insect chemosterilant isolated from *Acorus calamus.* London. *Nature* 270:512–513. (A biological insecticide.)

Saxena, D. B. et al. 1991. Fungi-toxicity of chemical components and some derivatives from *Anethum sowa* and *Acorus calamus. Indian Perfumery* 34(3):199–203. (Chemical compounds in the oil.)

Sharma, J. D. and P. C. Dandiya. 1962. Studies on *Acorus calamus* Part VI. Pharmacological actions of asarone and Beta-asarone on cardiovascular system and smooth muscles. *Indian J. Med. Res.* 50(1):61–65.

Siddiqui, M. T. A. and M. Asif. 1990. Anti-inflammatory activity of *Acorus calamus* L. (Abstract) New Delhi: *Conf. Pharmacol. Symp. on Herbal Drugs. 23.*

Vohora, S. B. et al. 1990 Central nervous system studies on an alcohol extract of *Acorus calamus* rhizomes. *J. Ethnopharmacol.* 28(1)53–62.

Vohora, S. B. et al. 1991. Antibacterial, antipyretic, analgesic and anti-inflammatory studies on *Acorus calamus* Linn. *Ann. Nat. Acad. Med. Sci.* 25(1)13–20. (The drug under trial conditions.)

4

Vasaka

Adhatoda vasica

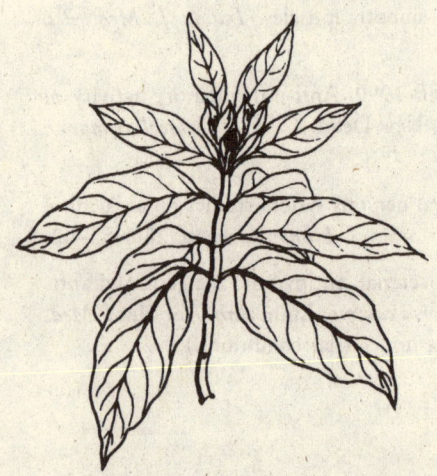

With vasaka the tongue
which knows no song will
learn to sing.

—A Tamil song from
Agasthyar

Passage to the Heavens

Vasaka grows in abundance in the lower reaches of the Himalayas,
where one often encounters several groups of sadhus practising
pranayama—a set of yogic breathing exercises. They occasionally
pluck and chew vasaka leaf-buds, usually with some ginger. They
believe that the drug cleans and clears the respiratory passage
and maintains their lungs and trachea in conditions healthy
enough to withstand their vigorous yogic sessions.

A passage to the Heavens may be painfully long, but vasaka
can ensure its smoothness!

Unrecognized Potential

Vasaka is indigenous, growing in the wilderness. Sometimes it is cultivated as a hedge-plant. Poor farmers often collect the twigs and leaves of this wild plant for use as green manure.

The drug vasaka comes from the fresh or dried leaves of the plant, and is known to destroy germs and worms. The drug is administered in the form of juice, syrup or decoction, and works by liquefying thickened sputum and facilitating its expulsion from the body.

Laboratory experiments conducted at the Haffkine Institute, Bombay are reported to have revealed that vasicinone, the alkaloid in vasaka, exhibits very powerful bronchodilator activity. It produces antitussive, anticonvulsant and antiarrhythmic activities thus confirming the tribal and traditional use of this drug in all types of respiratory disorders.

Profile

Botanical Names	:	*Adhatoda vasica* Nees	
		Adhatoda zeylanica Medik.	
		Justicia adhatoda Linn.	
English Name	:	Vasaka.	
Indian Names	:	Assamese	: *Bahaka, Herbuksha, Teeshae*
		Bengali	: *Vasaka*
		Gujarati	: *Alduso, Ardusi*
		Hindi	: *Adalsa, Adusa, Bansa, Vasika*
		Kannada	: *Adsele, Adusoge*
		Malayalam	: *Adalodakam*
		Marathi	: *Adulsa*
		Sanskrit	: *Atarusa, Vasaka, Vasika*
		Tamil	: *Aadaathodai*
		Telugu	: *Adasaramu, Atarushamu.*

Family	:	Acanthaceae.
Appearance	:	Tall, dense, evergreen shrub. Leaves, large, lance-shaped, somewhat resembling mango leaves. Fruit, a capsule with 4 seeds. Flowers, white or purple.
Distribution	:	Common in the Indian plains and the lower Himalayan ranges.
Medicinal Parts	:	Leaves, roots, flowers and bark.
Ayurvedic Preparations	:	*Chyavanapraasam, Vaasaarishtam, Valiya Raasnaadi Kashaayam.*

In Tradition

AILMENT	PRESCRIPTION
❧ Anaemia, asthma, cancer, cold, cough, chest pain, phlegm	: Crush 1 tbsp leaves and boil in 2 cups of water till reduced to 1 cup. Add 1 tsp honey. Drink 1/2 cup twice a day for 40 days.
❧ Asthma	: Take 3 or 4 small leaf-buds and chew together with a small piece of ginger for 40 days.
	: Mix together 1/2 cup each of the juices of vasaka leaves, pudina leaves, ginger (after removing any sediment) and lime in a porcelain bowl. Add 1 cup ajwain and mix again. Leave out under the sun till the mixture is dried thoroughly. Powder and preserve in a glass jar. *Dosage:* 1/4 tsp powder with 1 tsp honey, twice daily for a month.

❧ Asthma : Smoke the dried leaves after rolling them up into a cigar.

❧ Blood in : Grind 1 tbsp leaves in some water and urine (haematuria) drink.

❧ Bronchitis, cough : Boil leaf juice and honey (2:1 ratio) till the mixture acquires a paste-like consistency. Take $1/2$ tsp thrice a day.

❧ Bronchitis, cough, : Chop 3 leaves finely and heat till fever charred along with a little honey in a new mud vessel. When it begins to give off a characteristic odour, add $1/2$ tsp liquorice and $1/4$ tsp long pepper, and then 3 teacups water. Boil until reduced to $11/2$ teacups. Take 2 tbsp twice a day.

: Soak a few leaves every day in a mud pot containing drinking water. Whenever thirsty, drink a glass of this water with a few drops of honey.

❧ Cancer : Mix 20 drops of the leaf juice with goat's milk. Drink this effervescent mixture daily in the morning for 40 days. (*Note*: Large doses can cause vomiting and irritation.)

❧ Cough : Boil 4 to 5 leaves in water; strain. Add 1 tbsp honey. This is a very effective cough syrup.

: Make a herbal decoction by mixing 1 tsp each adhatoda leaves, black raisins and chebulic myrobalan in 2 cups

31

boiling water until reduced to $1/2$ cup.
Add sugar to taste and sip.

❧ Cough : Soak a few sticks of the roots of *kantakari* and adhatoda leaves in a mud pot containing drinking water. Whenever thirsty add a dash of long pepper and drink.

: See recipe for cough syrup below.

❧ Cough, fever, *kapha*-aggravation, phlegm : Cut 3 leaves and soak with one crushed cardamom in 3 cups water for 2 hours. Take 2 tbsp of this infusion three times a day.

❧ Diarrhoea, dysentery : 10 to 15 drops of the leaf juice administered once or twice a day.

❧ Eye diseases : Fry some flowers in a little ghee. Allow to cool. Apply on closed eyes and wrap with a napkin. Allow it to remain 15–20 minutes.

❧ Fever due to *pitta* or *vata* aggravation, phlegm : Boil 1 cup of the leaf juice in a mud pot till it acquires a paste-like consistency. Add 1 tsp ground long pepper. Take $1/2$ tsp thrice a day.

❧ Fever, jaundice : Extract 10 to 20 drops of the leaf juice. Mix with 1 tsp honey. Take once or twice a day.

❧ Intestinal worms : Mix 1 tsp ginger juice with a decoction of bark and root (10 to 20 drops). Take twice a day for 2–3 days.

32

❖ Liver problems : Extract 2 tsp juice from 2 or 3 leaves. Add 1 tsp honey. Take after breakfast.

❖ Slimy stools : Take 1 tsp of the leaf juice with $1/2$ cup curds in the morning.

❖ Swellings : Boil the leaves thoroughly in water (1:8 ratio) till the water is reduced to $1/8$ of the original volume. When bearably hot, soak a length of cloth in it and apply on the affected parts.

❖ Swellings, wounds : Warm the leaves over a flame and apply on the affected parts when bearably hot.

❖ Tuberculosis : Take 10 to 20 drops of the leaf juice with 1 tsp honey thrice a day.

: Take 2 tsp Vasaka Gulkand twice a day (Recipe below).

Note: Individual results may vary.

A Word of Caution

Vasaka in excess can cause severe vomiting.

Vasaka Cough Syrup

Cook 2 cups juice of fresh leaves of vasaka with 4 tbsp ghee and 1 cup sugar till the mixture acquires a syrupy consistency. Remove from heat and add $1/2$ tsp powdered long pepper.

Cool the mixture and add 1 cup honey. *Dosage:* 1 tbsp twice a day. *Note:* In the hot summer months, less long pepper is recommended as it tends to heat up the body.

Vasaka Gulkand

Vasaka Gulkand is used by traditional practitioners to treat tuberculosis. Take a handful of the fresh flowers. Crush them and sprinkle sugar crystals over them. Put out in a china bowl under the sun. Stir this mixture every morning and evening. After 4 weeks the preserve is ready to be used as complementary medicine.

Dose: $1/2$ to 1 tsp with warm milk.

In Science

Amin, A. H. 1961. Chemical and pharmacological studies of Vasicinone— A new alkaloid from *Adhatoda vasica* Nees. *Indian J. Pharma* 23:117. (Experimental verification: bronchial problems resolved; blood pressure in dogs brought down; coronary vessels in guinea-pigs and rabbits show increased flow.)

Bhatnagar, A. K. and S. P. Popli. 1966. Mass fragmentation of the alkaloids of *Adhatoda vasica* Nees. *Indian J. Chem.* 4:291–292. (A study.)

Bhide, M. B. et al. 1974. Pharmacological studies on vasicinone. *Bull. Haff. Inst.* 2:6.

————. 1975. Studies on the comparative pharmacological evaluation of vasicine and vasicinone. Ahmedabad: *All India Ayurvedic Scientific Seminar.*

————. 1980. Indigenous drugs in bronchial asthma. Simla: *Ann. Conf. of College of Allergy and Applied Immunology.* (Effective intervention in bronchial asthma.)

Bhide, M. B. and P. Y. Naik. 1977. Antiasthmatic potential of indigenous drug. Jamnagar: *Ayurvedic Research Seminar on Respiratory Diseases.* (Efficacy against asthma.)

————. 1980. Anti-asthmatic potentiality of vasicinone—an alkaloid from *Adhatoda vasica* Nees. Abstract. Bangkok: *Proc. of Asian Sym. in Med. Plants and Species.*

Chaturvedi, G. N. et al. 1983. Clinical trial of *Adhatoda vasica* syrup (*vasa*) in the patients of non-ulcer dyspepsia (amlapitta). *Anc. Sci. Life* 3(1):19–23. (Clinical confirmation of a folk practice.)

Chopra, R. N. et al. 1956. *Glossary of Indian Medicinal Plants.* New Delhi: CSIR. 7. (Use in rheumatism and bronchial asthma.)

Dhar, K. L. et al. 1981. Vasicol, a new alkaloid from *Adhatoda vasica. Phytochemistry* 20:319–321.

Doshi, J. J. et al. 1983. Effect of *Adhatoda vasica* massage in pyorrhoea. *Int. Jour. Crude Drug Res.* 21(4):173–176.

Gupta, O. P. et al. 1978. Vasicine alkaloid of *Adhatoda vasica,* a promising uterotonic abortifacient. *Indian J. Exp. Biol.* 16(10):1075–1077. (Anti-fertility role.)

Gupta, V. K. et al. 1983. Studies on the toxicity of vasicine hydrochloride on *Puntius sophere* and *Cyprinus carpio. Nat. Acad. Sci. Lett.* 6(7):239–241.

Jain, M. P. 1983. Vasaka, an Ayurvedic plant. *Science Rep.* 26(6):350–357. (A survey of vasaka.)

Jain, M. P. et al. 1980. Novel nor-harmal alkaloid from *Adhatoda vasica. Phytochemistry* 19:1880-1882.

Jain, M. P. and V. K. Sharma. 1982. Phytochemical investigation of root of *Adhatoda vasica. Planta Med.* 46:250.

Lahiri, P. K. and S. N. Pradhan. 1964. Pharmacological investigation of Vasicinol—an alkaloid from *Adhatoda vasica* Nees. *Indian J. Exp. Biol.* 2:219–223.

Pandita, K. et al. 1983. Seasonal variations of the alkaloids of *Adhatoda vasica* and detection of glycoside and n-oxides of vasicine and vasicinone. *Planta Med.* 48:65–128.

HOME REMEDIES

Sairam, T. V. 1997. Adhatoda. *Dignity Dialogue* 3(8): 31–39.

Shah, A. C. et al. 1987. A double-blind study of 'Wintry', a new broncho-dilator in asthmatic bronchitis. *Indian Pract*. 34(3):199–203. (Vasicine and vasicinone extracted from *Adhatoda zeylanica* are good for asthmatic bronchitis.)

Sharma, M. L. and C. K. Atal. 1985. Oxytocic, thrombopoietic and broncho-dilatory activities of vasicine—a novel molecule isolated from *Adhatoda vasica* Nees. Bombay: *Workshop on Selected Medicinal Plants used in Traditional/Indigenous Systems of Medicine*.

5

Aloe
Aloe vera

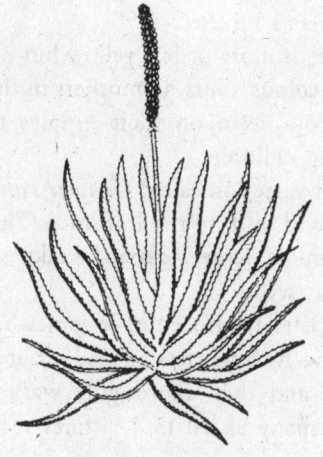

*Ghritakumari, cooling, bitter
. . . a fighter of pitta.*

—Raja Nighantu

Cosmetic Panacea

One of the most common ingredients in many a beauty product surprisingly comes from an unsightly plant that bears fierce-looking thorns: aloe. The plant is called the Virgin (*kumari* in Sanskrit), as it offers a new lease of life and possibilities for rejuvenation and renewal.

Egyptian history refers to the aloe as a favourite herb in Cleopatra's toilette. It is the pulp of the plant which is known for its cosmetic as well as medicinal importance.

Succour of the Poor

The aloe has been used widely not only by the rich and famous, but also by the poor who suffer silently from various ailments. The Kotas in the Nilgiris remove the spines and peel off the leaves to obtain the fleshy pulp, which is used to treat rheumatic joints.

The Gonds of Madhya Pradesh commonly use the fleshy leaves to heal wounds. The leaf is longitudinally but partially split and bandaged over wounds and injuries.

The fresh juice from the leaves is more or less yellow but on drying acquires a brownish black colour. Nursing mothers in the villages apply this yellow, nauseous resin on their nipples to make them distasteful to weaning children.

Unani practitioners prepare a confection called *Ganwar Pathe ka Halwa* by adding ghee, sugar and milk to the leaf juice. This preparation is administered as a tonic to remedy general weakness. It is believed to be aphrodisiac as well.

The pulp is quite bitter to taste. It also emits a somewhat offensive smell. In order to remove its bitterness and odour, it is often sliced into very thin bits and then thoroughly washed repeatedly in running water, as many as 10 to 15 times. The resultant mass finds its use in several beauty preparations and indigenous medicines. Some native physicians also sun-dry the pulp, and a lustrous black, hard mass known variously as *alva*, *elua* and *masasaber* is obtained. Though bitter, it is palatable when diluted with water or apple juice. This is used as a reputed remedy for intestinal worms in children.

The drug is considered to be an effective tonic for stomach ailments; it is often combined with ajwain before administration. It is also considered useful in the maintenance of a healthy circulatory system, liver, spleen, and the female reproductive system.

The drug contains the active principle aloins, which is responsible for its purgative action.

Profile

Botanical Names	:	*Aloe vera* (Linn.) Burm. f. *Aloe barbadensis* Mill.
English Names	:	Aloe, Barbados Aloe, Curaçao Aloe, Indian Aloe, Jaffarabad Aloe.

Indian Names   :

Hindi	:	*Gheekanvar*
Malayalam	:	*Katavala, Kumari*
Tamil	:	*Kariyapolam, Musambaram, Sotrukatrazhai*
Telugu	:	*Chinnakalabanda*
Sanskrit	:	*Kumari*
Ayurvedic	:	*Ghrtakumari, Kumari*
Unani	:	*Gheekumar.*

Chinese Name	:	*Lu hui.*
Family	:	Liliaceae.
Appearance	·	The fibrous root produces a rosette of succulent, lance-like leaves, whitish-green on both sides with spines on the margin. Flowers, orange or yellow to purplish, in racemes. Fruit, a triangular capsule, ellipsoid-oblong.
Distribution	:	Introduced, now running wild throughout India. Common along the coasts of South East/West India.
Medicinal Parts	:	The mucilaginous gel-like pulp obtained on peeling the leaves and its dried form (powder); leaves.
Ayurvedic Formulations	:	*Kumaryasavam, Valiya Chandanadi Tailam, Annabhedi-Sinduram, Manjisthadi Tailam, Kumarika Vati, Kumari Paka, Rajah Parvatini Vati.*

39

Unani Preparations	:	*Sufuf Dama.*
Preparation and Dosage	:	Infusion (Dissolve 1 tsp aloe in 2 cups water along with 2 tsp boric acid); powder (*dosage*: 1 to 5 grains); extract (10 to 30 drops).
Other species	:	*Aloe latifolia.* (In South Africa, the leaf pulp is used for the treatment of boils, inflammations, ringworm and sores.) *Aloe tenuior.* (The decoction of the root is used to curb tapeworm infestation.) *Aloe saponaria.* (In South Africa, the leaf pulp is used for the treatment of ringworm.) *Aloe perryi.* (Also known as Bombay Aloe, it is also used the same way as Barbados Aloe, even though its potency is reportedly less.)

In Tradition

AILMENT		PRESCRIPTION
❧ Blood-dysentery	:	Grind $1/10$ tsp of pulp along with cumin seeds and sugar candy and eat.
❧ Blood in urine, burning sensation during urination	:	Swallow $1/10$ tsp of washed pulp every morning for a week.
❧ Boils, pimples	:	Crush the leaves and apply the paste locally for a few days.
❧ Boils, skin-eruptions	:	Bandage the affected areas with the pulp.

❧ Burns, cuts,
insect bites, itch,
scratches, wrinkles
: Split the fresh leaves and expose the fresh juice to the sun for a while and then rub on the affected parts.

❧ Burns, herpes, sores : Apply fresh juice on the affected areas.

❧ Cold, cough
: Roast the leaf and extract the juice. Take $1/2$ tsp in 1 cup warm water.

❧ Constipation,
gas
: Take 2 tsp aloe oil (Recipe below) at bedtime.

❧ Convulsions,
excessive thirst
: Warm the leaf-gel and take $1/10$ tsp.

❧ Diarrhoea
: Take $1/2$ tsp of the leaf-paste and mix into it 1 tsp each cumin powder and sugar candy. Take once or twice.

❧ Fatigue
: Take $1/10$ tsp gel with a pinch of turmeric powder.

❧ Fatigue, senility
: Dry the leaves and powder. Take 5 grains of the fine powder every day with food.

❧ Goitre
: Grind equal quantities of ajwain, borax and turmeric. Mix 1 tsp of the finely ground mixture with 1 tbsp aloe pulp. Heat slightly and apply gently on the affected parts.

❧ Hair loss,
insomnia
: Boil a mixture of equal quantities of leaf juice and gingelly oil till all moisture has evaporated. Apply on the head and massage for a few minutes before retiring.

❧ Irritation in the eyes

: Dissolve $1/2$ tsp aloe and 1 tsp boric acid in 1 cup water. Use the solution as an eyewash. (*Caution:* Take all hygiene measures to prevent infection.)

❧ Itch, prolapsed rectum, scanty urination

: Expel the juice and mix into it some butter, powder of tail pepper and sugar candy. Eat it.

: Remove the thorns in the margin of the leaf and split it into two halves. Gently warm over a charcoal fire and sprinkle on them finely powdered chebulic myrobalan. Bandage these treated leaf halves on the prolapsed mass.

❧ Redness of eyes

: Scoop out the pulp and bandage over the eyelids before going to bed. Repeat for 3 days.

❧ Rheumatism

: Warm the pulp and apply on the affected areas.

❧ Stomach ache, ulceration

: Boil $1/2$ cup sugar candy, $1/2$ cup small onions (cut into small pieces), $1/4$ cup sliced pulp in $1/2$ cup castor oil till the mixture achieves a jam-like consistency. Cool and bottle. *Dose*: 1 tsp twice a day.

❧ Swelling

: Mix the pulp in water and boil. Use as poultice.

❧ Swelling, injuries, wounds

: Dissolve 1 tbsp extracted juice of aloe in $1/2$ cup hot water and apply on the affected area.

❖ Wounds   : Split the leaf longitudinally and partially
                           and use to bandage the wounds.

Note: Individual results may vary.

A Word of Caution

Aloe is a powerful laxative. It must be used with great caution.
Aloe causes nausea and hence it is desirable to combine it with
more palatable substances like ajwain, apple juice, etc. It can
cause serious griping and hence it is advisable to take it with
carminatives like turmeric or rose petals.

Aloe Oil

The pulp of aloe has a nauseating smell and taste and hence
cannot be used as such. Traditionally, it is made into an oil in
the following manner:

Fleshy leaves are selected and their outer skin and spines are
removed carefully with the help of a sharp knife. The fleshy pulp
is now cut into small bits and then washed thoroughly in running
water at least 10 to 15 times. Pat dry in a thick dry towel. Place
1 cup of the dry bits in a wide-mouthed saucepan and add 2
cups pure castor oil, 1 cup powdered palm candy and $1/4$ cup
sliced white onions. Heat well over a low flame till the last traces
of moisture in the oil have evaporated. Cool and bottle. *Dose*: 1
tsp twice a day for stomach disorders, loss of appetite, ulceration
in the stomach and the intestines, stomach ache, gastritis, etc.

In Science

Ahmed, S. et al. 1990. Aloe—a biologically active and potential
medicinal plant. *Hamdard Medicus* 36(1):108–115. (A monograph.)

Ajab Noor, M. A. 1991. Effect of Aloe on blood glucose levels in normal and alloxan diabetic mice. *J. Ethnopharmacol.* 28(2):215–220. (Antidiabetic.)

Awe, W. and H. J. Kuemmel. 1962. Aloe. VII. The presence of aloin in *Aloe vera* and comparative investigation with a fresh sample of Cape Aloe (*Aloe ferox*) and prepared dry extract therefrom. *Arch. Pharm.* 295:819.

Bhandari, C. R. and B. Mukerji. 1959. Aloes. *Pharmaceutist* 5:39.

Central Council for Research in Ayurveda and Siddha. 1996. *Pharmacological Investigations of Certain Medicinal Plants and Compound Formulations used in Ayurveda and Siddha.* New Delhi. 108–111. (Anti-ulcerogenic and hypotensive.)

Cera, L. M. et al. 1980. The therapeutic efficacy of *Aloe vera* cream (Dermaide Aloe) in thermal injuries (2 cases). *J. Am. Anim. Hosp. Assoc.* 16(5):768–772; *Biol. Abstr.* 71:83007. 1981. (Bactericidal and antiprostaglandin effect.)

Chopra, R. N. and N. N.Ghosh. 1938. Chemical examination of Indian Aloes. *Arch. Pharm.* 34B:276.

Chopra, R. N. et al. 1956. *Glossary of Indian Medicinal Plants.* New Delhi: Council of Scientific and Industrial Research 13. (Use of *aloe* in menstrual disorders.)

Chowdhury, R. R. et al. 1980. Review of plants screened for anti-fertility activity III. *Bull. Medico-Ethno-Bot. Res.* 1(4):542–545.

Dixit, P. and H. C. Jain. 1985. Anti-arteriosclerotic factor of *Aloe barbedense* ethanolic extract in dogs. *Adv. Biosci.* 4(1):95–99. (Anti-arteriosclerotic activity.)

Elizabeth, R. and A. J. Haagen Smit. 1948. Mucilage from *Aloe vera.* *J. Amer. Chem. Soc.* 70:3248.

Frawley, D. and V. Lad. 1994. *The Yoga of Herbs—An Ayurvedic Guide to Herbal Medicine.* Delhi: Motilal Banarsidas.

Goswami, C. S. and M. M. Bokadia. 1979. Effect of extracts of *Aloe barbadensis* Mill. leaves on fertility of female rats. *Indian Drugs* 16(6):124–125. (Anti-fertility activity of the plant.)

Gottshall, R. Y. et al. 1950. Antibacterial substances in seed plants active against Tubercle bacilli. *Ann. Rev. Tuberculosis.* 62:475. (The plant inhibits the growth of *Mycobacterium tuberculosis.*)

Gupta, K. 1972. Aloe compound (a herbal drug) in functional sterility XVI. *Obst. Gyna. Cong.* New Delhi. (Improvement of fertility.)

Joshi, C. G and N. G. Nagar. 1952. Antibiotic activity of some Indian medicinal plants. *J. Sci. Industr. Res.* 11B(6):261. (The plant's role in fighting the bacteria: *E. coli* and *S. aureus.*)

Katoka, M. and Y. Takagaki. 1992. Screening of crude drugs having anti-allergic effect using ratbasophilic leukaemia cells. *Shoyakugaku Zasshi.* 46(1):25–29. (Controls allergy.)

Khan, S. S. and D. Malhotra. 1996. Indian Medicinal Plants III. *Aloe vera* L. *Acta Clinica Scientica* 5 & 6 (I& II) 57–59.

Kurup, P. N. V. et al. 1979. *Handbook of Medicinal Plants.* New Delhi. 125. (In hair-regeneration.)

Lushbangh, C. C. and B. B. Hale. 1953. Experimental acute radio determination following y-irradiation V. Histopathological study of mode of action of therapy with *Aloe vera. Cancer* 6:690.

Map, P. K. and T. J. McCarthy. 1970. Assessment of purgative principles in Aloes. *Planta Med.* 19:361.

Marrow, D. M. et al. 1981. Hyper-sensitivity to Aloe. *Arch. Dermatol* 116(9):1064–1065; *Biol. Abstr.* 71:7229.

Moosa, J. S. 1985. A study on the crude anti-diabetic drugs used in Arabian folk-medicine. *Int. J. Crude Drug Res.* 23(3):137–145. (Significant hypoglycaemic activity in experimental mice.)

Nadkarni, A. K. 1954. *Indian Materia Medica.* Bombay. 74. (Cures dyspepsia, flatulence, intestinal colic, dysuria and general debility.)

Rowe, T. D. 1940. Effect of *Aloe vera* gel in the treatment of third degree Roentgen reactions on white rats. A preliminary report. *J. Amer. Pharm. Assn.* 29:348.

———. 1941. A phytochemical study of *Aloe vera* leaf. *J. Amer. Pharm. Assn.* 30:262.

Sairam, T. V. 1998. Aloe Vera. *Dignity Dialogue*, May 16–17.

Singh, M. et al. 1973. Beneficial effects of *Aloe vera* with healing of thermal burns and radiation injury in albino rats. *Indian J. Pharmac.* 5:258. (The expressed juice of aloe in the form of an ointment in vaseline hastens the healing process in thermal burns and radiation injuries.)

Sivarajan, V. V. and I. Balachandran. 1994. *Ayurvedic Drugs and their Plant Sources*. New Delhi: Oxford & IBH. 261–262. (Usefulness in haemophilia, skin and uterine disorders, liver and spleen enlargement, eye infections, painful swellings, chronic ulcers and disorders due to the aggravation of *kapha* and *pitta*.)

Sharma, P. V. 1983. *Dravyaguna Vigyana*. Varanasi. 449. (Aloe fights cough.) (In Hindi.)

Sharma, S. C. et al. 1972. The effect of *Aloe indica* on the fertility of female rabbits XVI. New Delhi: Indian Obst. Gyna. Congress. (Fertility and implantation properties.)

Shinpo, M. et al. 1978. Anti-inflammatory compositions containing *Aloe* extracts and steroids. *Japan Kokai* 78, 49, 019; *Chem. Abstr.* 89:95018m. (Anti-inflammatory use.)

Thyagarajan, R. et al. 1977. Studies with Siddha drugs in infective hepatitis. *J. Res. Indian Med. Yoga & Homoeo.* 12(2):1. (Protective effect on patients with infective hepatitis and hepato-toxicity.)

Waller, G. R. et al. 1978. Natural products from *Aloe barbadensis* Miller. *Lloydia* 41:648.

6

Galangal

Alpinia galanga

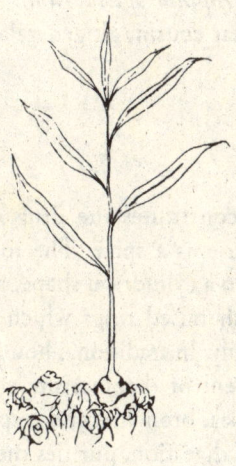

> *Destroyer of kapha and vata.*
>
> —Bhava Prakasa Nighantu

Herb of Yore

Galangal is believed to have come from Java. However the Arabian geographer Ibn Khurdabah (9th Century A.D.) associated it with Sila, present-day China.

Plutarch the Greek essayist (1st Century A.D.) records that the ancient Egyptians had used this plant as a fumigating spice.

Marco Polo the Venetian traveller (13th Century A.D.) has also recorded numerous references to this spice in his travelogues.

Charaka the great compiler of the treatise on Ayurveda (2nd Century B.C.) included Galangal in the category of drugs that are capable of imparting youthful vigour and strength.

The plant has for as yet inexplicable reasons fallen into disuse in most parts of the globe, the only exceptions being India and Russia.

The Galangal Family

A more apposite name, Greater Galangal was coined to distinguish it from its cousin, Lesser Galangal (*Alpinia officinarum*).

Like yet another but more popular cousin, ginger, galangal is also an aromatic stimulant.

The Drug

The dried rootstock of this plant constitutes the drug. In the historical past, it was in common use as a spice. The roots are often cut while they are still fresh into a cylindrical shape, marked at short intervals by narrow, whitish raised rings which help a native doctor to identify the drug easily. In traditional households, the drug finds its use in the treatment of rheumatism, stomach disorders, flatulence, dyspepsia, nausea, bronchial and respiratory complaints in children. It stimulates digestion, purifies the blood and improves the timbre of the voice.

It is the acrid resin and volatile oils found in the rootstock that make it medicinal. It also contains tannins and flavonoids.

Galangal Oil, which is referred to as False Ginger Oil, is a pale yellow to olive brown liquid with an eucalyptus-cardamom-ginger-like smell and a bitter taste.

Recent clinical investigations of the drug reveal its remarkable efficacy. Intravenous injections of a small dose of its infusion have produced a sharp fall in blood pressure in experimental animals. In a short time however, the blood pressure returns to normal. The fall in blood pressure is reportedly due to dilation of the blood vessels. Some Japanese scientists have isolated two anti-tumour principles from this plant.

The Arabs feed the drug to their horses to keep them in fine fettle.

Profile

Botanical Names	:	*Alpinia galanga* (L) Willd. *Languas galanga* (L) Stuntz.
English Names	:	Galangal, Greater Galangal, Java Galangal.

Indian Names :

Bengali	: *Kulanjan*
Gujarati	: *Kolinjan*
Hindi	: *Kalanjan, Kulinjan, Punnagchampa, Sugandhbach*
Kannada	: *Rasmi, Sugandha Vachi, Dumparasme, Doddarasagadde*
Malayalam	: *Aratta, Peraratta*
Marathi	: *Baripankijar, Koshikulinjan, Koshtakulinjan*
Punjabi	: *Kulanjan*
Sanskrit	: *Kulanja, Kulanjana, Rasna, Sugandhamula*
Sindhi	: *Kathi, Kunjar*
Tamil	: *Aratai, Peraratai*
Telugu	: *Dumparastramu, Kachoramu, Peddadumparashtrakamu*
Urdu	: *Kulanjan*
Ayurvedic	: *Kulanjana, Rasna.*

Family	:	Zingiberaceae.
Appearance	:	About 2 metres tall, a perennial herb with an aromatic rootstock. Smooth leaf sheaths

	cover the lower portion of the plant. Flowers, faintly fragrant, pale greenish-white. Fruits, deep orange-red in colour. Seeds, 3-angled, ash-coloured and pungent.
Distribution	: Found in the Eastern Himalayas and South West India.
Medicinal Parts	: Rhizome (Rootstock).
Ayurvedic Preparations	: As anti-inflammatory decoctions: *Rasna Adikamath, Rasna Saptak Kwath.* Others: *Rasnadi Kashayam, Rasnadi Churnam, Rasnadi Tailam, Ashwagandharishtam.*
Unani Preparations	: As aphrodisiac preparations: *Ma'jun Mugawivi Ma Mumsik, Ma'jun Samagh.* As antispasmodic tonic: *Ma'jun Chobchini, Lubab Mo'tadil.* As a cardiac stimulant: *Arq Pan.*
Other Species	: *Alpinia calacrata* (*Perarattai* in Tamil) and *Alpinia officinarun* (Lesser Galangal) exhibit properties similar to the Greater Galangal.

In Tradition

AILMENT	PRESCRIPTION
❧ Asthma, chest congestion, cough, phlegm	: Crush $1/2$ tsp rootstock and soak in a pot of drinking water (2 cups) for 3–4 hours. Drink the infusion after adding to it 1 tsp honey.
❧ Bad breath, throat-irritation	: Crush a bit of the rootstock and chew with betel leaf.

✤ Cold, cough, : Powder roughly equal quantities of the
 fever, headache,   rootstock and sugar candy separately
 lung diseases,   and then mix the powders together.
 nausea, pneumonia Take 1/2 tsp with hot water or milk.

✤ Cold, cough, : Crush 1 tsp each of galangal, long
 fever, headache,   pepper, liquorice and talispatri
 phlegm   (*Flacourtia cataphracta*) with a little
           water and grind well. Heat this paste
           in 4 teacups water till it comes to the
           boil. Filter. Take 1 teacup of this
           decoction along with 1 tsp honey thrice
           daily.

         : Soak a pea-sized rhizome in 1 cup
           boiling water for 3 hours. Filter. Add 1
           tbsp palm sugar. *Dose:* 3 tbsp thrice
           daily.

✤ Cough, nausea : Dip a rhizome in castor oil and show
           over a naked flame till it is charred.
           Powder and store. *Dose:* 1/4 to 1/2 tsp
           with honey.

✤ Cough, nausea, : Crush a small piece of the rootstock
 phlegm   along with sugar candy and eat.

✤ Gum infections : Gargle with the infusion frequently.

✤ Phlegm-accumula- : Drop a small piece of crushed
 tion, throat-   galangal in 3 cups of boiling water
 congestion, *pitta*- and allow it to infuse for 3 to 4 hours.
 aggravation   Filter and add 2 tbsp sugar candy. Take
           2 tbsp thrice a day.

Note: Individual results may vary.

In Science

Chopra, I. C. et al. 1957. Antibacterial properties of volatile principles of *Alpinia galanga* and *Acorus calamus*. *Antibiotics Chemother*. 7:378. (Stimulation of the bronchial glands occurs on exposure to the oil-vapours.)

Chunekar, K. C. 1982. *Bhavaprakasanighantu of Sri Bhavamisra*. Commentary. Varanasi. (The action of galangal in stimulating digestion, purifying the blood and improving the voice.) (In Hindi)

Inamdar, M. C. et al. 1961. Expectorant activity of *Alpinia galanga*. *Indian J. Physiol. Pharmacol.* 6:150. (The volatile oil as a carminative.)

Itokawa, H. et al. 1987. Antitumor principles from *Alpinia galanga*. *Planta Med.* 53(1):32–33. (Isolation of two antitumour principles from the plant.)

Pruthi, J. S. 1976. *Spices and Condiments*. New Delhi: National Book Trust. 122.

Sairam, T. V. 1998. Greater Galangal. *Dignity Dialogue*, June 20–21.

Sastry, M. S. 1961. Comparative chemical study of two varieties of galangal. *Indian J. Pharm.* 23:76.

Thakur, R. S. et al. 1989. *Medicinal Plants of India*. Lucknow: CIMAP.

7

Devil's Tree

Alstonia scholaris

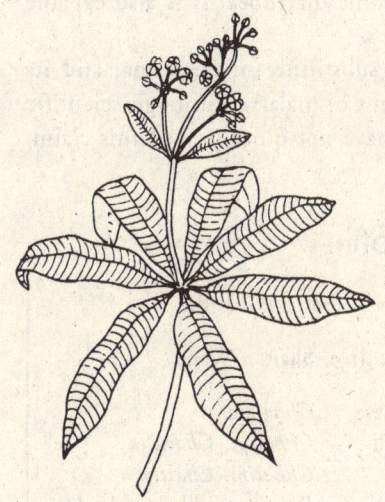

Saptaparna, a remedy for ulcers with foul discharges.

—Kaiya Deva Nighantu

The Devil's Due

In Indian mythology, gods are often associated with flora. While tulsi is considered the abode of the Goddess of Wealth, Lakshmi, bel represents the three-eyed Lord Shiva, durva grass the elephant-headed Ganesha, amla the God of Wealth, Kubera and so on. When gods can have their favourite flora then why not the devil? The answer, of course, is the Devil's Tree! The name of the tree is evidently from folk beliefs and tales that associate this tree with evil: the tribes in the Western Ghats avoid even passing by this tree for fear of its malefic properties.

Despite its name, this tropical tree, distinguished by seven leaves in a whorl and a very bitter milky leaf juice seems to be quite considerate towards humankind.

The medicinal bark is pale ash-grey in colour. It is commercially recognized as ditta bark. It is a sought-after remedy for fevers in Santhal households. It is also a recognized remedy for several skin ailments: acne, eczema and ringworm. Besides, it is used in the treatment of chronic diarrhoea. It is also capable of destroying intestinal parasites.

The drug is used too as a substitute for cinchona, and its alkaloid, quinine in the treatment of malaria, although scientific experiments conducted so far have not quite proved this claim.

Profile

Botanical Name	:	*Alstonia scholaris* (L) R.Br.	
English Names	:	Devil's Tree, Shaitan Wood.	
Indian Names	:	Assamese	: *Chhaiten*
		Bengali	: *Chhatim, Chatwan*
		Hindi	: *Chhatim, Chattiyan, Saptparna, Shaitan ka Jat*
		Kannada	: *Hale, Maddale*
		Malayalam	: *Daivapala, Elilampala, Pala, Yakshi Pala*
		Marathi	: *Satvin, Shaitan*
		Oriya	: *Chatiana*
		Sanskrit	: *Saptaparna*
		Tamil	: *Elilaipalai, Palai*
		Telugu	: *Edakulapala, Phalagaruda*
		Urdu	: *Satoona*
		Sanskrit	: *Saptaparna*
		Unani	: *Satoona.*
Family	:	Apocynaceae.	

Appearance	:	An evergreen tree with milky juice. Bark, pale, ash-grey in colour. Leaves, leathery, dark green on dorsal side, oblong-lance-like. In whorls of 4 to 7. Flowers, greenish-white in terminal clusters, spice-scented. Fruit, hanging in pairs. The fruit contain hairy seeds.
Distribution	:	Tropical and deciduous forests of India.
Medicinal Parts	:	Bark, milky juice, root. *Dose:* 1 to 2 tsp decoction along with 1 to 2 tsp honey twice a day.

In Tradition

AILMENT	PRESCRIPTION
❧ Catarrhal dyspepsia, gastritis, mucus in stools	: Mix $1/2$ tsp finely powdered ditta bark in boiling water and leave to infuse for an hour. Drink the infusion at bedtime.
❧ Diarrhoea, fatigue after illness	: Soak 3 tsp bark powder in $2^1/_2$ teacups : boiling water for 1 hour. Filter and drink 1 to 2 tbsp 2–3 times a day.
❧ Fever, gastritis, intestinal worms, pain in testicles, phlegm, rheumatism, scrotal hernia	: Grind the root into a very fine powder. Take $1/4$ tsp along with 1 teacup hot water.
❧ Headache, rheumatic pain, ulcers with foul discharges	: Grind the bark and dilute with a little water. Warm and apply as a plaster and bandage tightly.

: Extract the milky juice from the plant and apply externally on the affected areas.

: Apply tender leaves as a poultice.

In Science

Bakhru, H. K. 1992. *Herbs that Heal—Natural Remedies for Good Health.* Delhi: Orient Paperbacks. (Divinity in the devil's tree.)

Bodding, P. O. 1986. Studies in Santhal medicine and connected folklore. Parts I, II and III. Calcutta: The Asiatic Society. (The bark cures headaches.)

Chakravarty, D. et al. 1954. Examination of Ditta bark. *Bull. Calcutta Sch. Trop. Med. Hyg.* 2:4. (Chemistry of the bark.)

———. 1955. Chemical examination of Ditta bark. Part II. *Bull. Calcutta. Sch. Trop. Med. Hyg.* 3:4. (The alkaloids of the bark.)

———. 1956. Chemical examination of Ditta bark. Part III. *Bull. Calcutta Sch. Trop. Med. Hyg.* 4:4. (The identification of alkaloids.)

Chatterjee, A. et al. 1965. The alkaloids of the leaves of *Alstonia scholaris* R. Br. *Tetrahedron Lett.* 41:3633. (Chemical composition of the leaves.)

———. 1978. Alkaloids of *Alstonia venenata* E.Br. *J. Scient. Industr. Res.* 37:187. (*Alstonia venenata*, a related species is reported to contain 24 bases.)

Dhar, M. L. et al. 1968. Screening of Indian plants for biological activity. Part I. *Indian J. Exp. Biol.* 6:232. (The alkaloids as crude extract were ineffective against malaria; however, they gave low hypotensive activity.)

Rastogi, R. C. et al. 1970. Picralinal, a key alkaloid of picralimin group from *Alstonia scholaris* R. Br. *Experientia* 26:1956.

Talapatra, R. P. et al. 1967. Isolation of echitamine chloride from the root and root bark of *Alstonia scholaris* R. Br. *J. Indian Chem. Soc.* 44:639. (Chemistry of the alkaloids.)

8

Indian Birthwort

Aristolochia indica

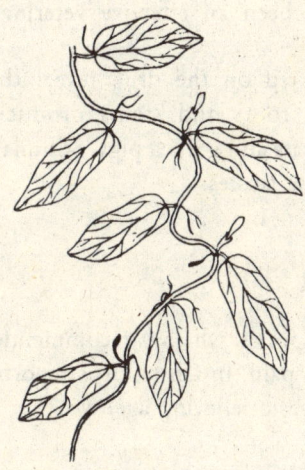

Ishwari conquers every type of toxin and leprosy too.

—Hrdayapriya

The Great Antidote

Almost all the names of this plant in ancient Sanskrit literature focus entirely on its capacity as an antidote to all maner of poisons: *Nakuli, Garudi, Karalakah, Visaghni, Visavega,* for instance. Forest-dwellers in India have long known about this plant and have been using it particularly in the treatment of snakebite.

Curiously, the tribal practice of using this plant to treat snakebite draws inspiration from the peculiar shape of the flower which bears a strong resemblance to a cobra's hood.

Ayurveda has endorsed this folk tradition; it considers the root bark a very effective antidote to snake-poison.

In tribal pockets, the fresh juice of the leaves and also of the bark is commonly used to treat bowel complaints in children, diarrhoea and intermittent fevers. The drug is believed to promote digestion and regulate menstruation, when administered in small doses. As it cleanses the impurities in the blood, it helps in curing deadly skin diseases such as leprosy.

The root bark has also long been an effective veterinary medicine.

Scientific experiments conducted on the drug reveal that alcoholic water extracts of the roots and stems produced contraction of the uteri in virgin rats and guinea pigs. Stimulant effects were also observed on these tissues.

The Chinese Aristolochia

Aristolochia debilis is the Chinese species, which is recommended for snakebite, throat and stomach pain, in China. It is reported to contain anti-tumour and analgesic relieving agents.

Profile

Botanical Name	: *Aristolochia indica* L.	
English Name	: Indian Birthwort.	
Indian Names	: Bengali	: *Isurmul*
	Gujarati	: *Arkmula, Sapsu*
	Hindi	: *Isharmul, Ishwari*
	Kannada	: *Eashwari-Beru*
	Malayalam	: *Gaudakodi, Ishwaramuli, Karalakam*
	Marathi	: *Sapasan*
	Oriya	: *Gopakaroni*

Sanskrit	: *Ishwari, Ishwarimul*
Tamil	: *Garudakodi, Isuramuli*
Telugu	: *Guntaganjeera, Iswaraveru*
Ayurvedic	: *Garudi, Isaramula*
Unani	: *Zarawend-i-Hind.*

Family : Aristolochiaceae.

Appearance : A twiner. Stems, woody in lower parts, but softer above. Leaves vary in size and shape, triple-nerved. Flowers, purple, trumpet-like in shape, resembling a cobra's hood. Fruit, a 6-valved capsule. Seeds flat and winged.

Distribution : Throughout India in the foothills and plains, particularly in the tract extending from Nepal to peninsular India through Bengal. Usually found spreading over hedges and bushes as wild growth.

Medicinal Parts : Dried stems and roots. *Dose:* 1 to 2 tsp powder along with 1 tsp honey twice a day. 1 to 2 tsp decoction twice a day.

Ayurvedic Preparations: *Parantyadi Tailam, Pathadi Gulika, Neeleedalaadi Tailam.*

Other species : *Aristolochia bracteolata* Lamk. Kiramar (H); Dhumrapatra (S). The root powder is used in the treatment of foul ulcers and worms.

In Tradition

AILMENT	PRESCRIPTION
♣ Catarrh, cough, diarrhoea, dyspepsia, fever, flatulence, intestinal worms, weakness of the heart	: Mix 1 tsp root powder along with 1/2 tsp pepper powder and take with 1 cup hot water.

❧ Cough, leprosy, : Powder the root. Take 1 tsp with
ulcers   1 tsp honey.

❧ Dyspepsia, digestive : Powder the root and take a pinch with
problems, inter-   warm water frequently.
mittent fevers

❧ Inflammations : Grind the seeds into a very fine paste
      with some water and apply locally.

❧ Leucoderma (initial : Apply a fine paste of leaves on the
stages), skin diseases, affected areas. Allow to dry.
swellings, wounds

Note: Individual results may vary.

In Science

Achari, B. et al. 1981. Studies on Indian medicinal plants. Part 63. An N-glycoside and steroids from *Aristolochia indica*. *Phytochemistry* 20:1444. (The plant steroids and their uses.)

——. 1982. Studies on Indian medicinal plants. Part 69: A new 4, 5-dioxo aporphine and other constituents of *Aristolochia indica*. *Heterocycles* 19:1203.

——. 1983. Studies on Indian medicinal plants. Part 72: A phenanthroid lactone, steroid and lignans from *Aristolochia indica*. *Heterocycles* 20:771. (Chemical constituents of the bark.)

——. 1984. Studies on Indian medicinal plants. Part 76. Carbon 13-NMR spectra of some phenanthrene derivatives from *Aristolochia indica* and their analogues. *Org. Magn. Reson.* 22:741.

Che, C. T. et al. 1984. Studies on *Aristolochia* III. Isolation and biological evaluation of constituents of *Aristolochia indica* roots for fertility-regulating activity. *J. Nat. Prod.* 47:331. (The plant lowers fertility, although certain individual compounds are not found effective in interrupting pregnancy.)

Dutta, M. K. and M. S. Sastry. 1959. Pharmacological action of *Aristolochia bracteata* Retz. on the uterus. *Indian J. Pharm.* 20:302. (100% interceptive activity and 91.7% anti-implantation activity constitute the findings of the data studied here.)

Fuehrer, H. et al. 1970. Ishwarone. *Tetrahedron* 26:2371.

Ganguly, A. K. et al. 1969. Ishwarone, a novel tetracyclic sesquiterpene. *Tetrahedron Lett.* 3:133.

Ganshirt, H. 1953. The isolation of aristolochic acid from various aristolochaceae and its quantitative derivation. *Pharmazie* 8:584.

Kupchan, S. M. and J. J. Merianos. 1968. Tumor inhibitors XXXII. Isolation and structural elucidation of novel derivatives of aristolochic acid from *Aristolochia indica*. *J. Org. Chem.* 33:3735.

Pakrashi, A. and B. Chakravarti. 1978. Antiestrogenic and anti-implantation effect of aristolic acid from *Aristolochia indica* Linn. *Indian J. Exp. Biol.* 16:1283 (Anti-estrogenic and anti-implantation effects in mice.)

Pakrashi, S. C. et al. 1977. Studies on Indian medicinal plants. Part 46. New phenanthrene derivatives from *Aristolochia indica*. *Phytochemistry* 16:1103.

———. 1980. Studies on Indian medicinal plants. Part 60: (125)-7, 12-secoiswaran-12-ol, a new type of sesquiterpene from *Aristolochia indica*. *J. Org. Chem.* 45:4765.

Pakrashi, S. C. and C. Saha. 1977. Effect of a sesquiterpene from *Aristolochia indica* Linn. on fertility in female mice. *Experientia* 1977. 33:1498.

Thakur, R. S. et al. 1989. *Major Medicinal Plants of India*. Lucknow.: CIMAP.

9

Shatavari

Asparagus racemosus

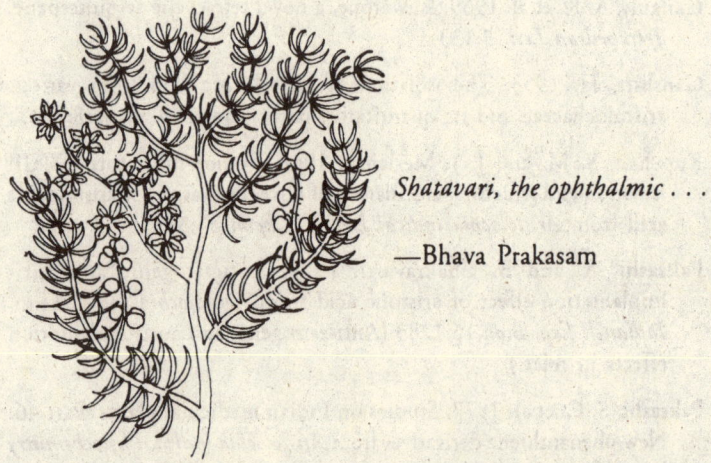

Shatavari, the ophthalmic . . .

—Bhava Prakasam

Food for Thought

In the rural areas, the fresh roots of shatavari, cleaned and chopped, are fed to buffaloes—this is believed to increase their milk-yield. It is also an important vegetable in the Kumaon hills. In Bangladesh, the blanched shoots are made into a preserve.

Shatavari is categorized in Ayurveda as a powerful *rasayana* drug, which can improve physical as well as mental performance by slowing down the ageing process. It is also a favourite galactagogue, which induces milk secretion in nursing mothers. It is widely used in the treatment of amoebiasis, diabetes, diarrhoea, dyspepsia and tumours.

Recent laboratory experiments as detailed elsewhere in this chapter have confirmed folk wisdom: the plant has been found to possess anti-amoebic, anti-ulcer, hypoglycaemic, anti-viral and anticancer properties!

Profile

Botanical Name	:	*Asparagus racemosus* Willd.
English Names	:	Sparrow-Grass, Wild Asparagus.
Indian Names	:	

Bengali	:	*Satamuli*
Gujarati	:	*Ekalkanto, Satavari*
Hindi	:	*Satamuli, Satvar, Shatavari*
Kannada	:	*Challagadda, Satamulike*
Malayalam	:	*Satavali, Nannari*
Marathi	:	*Asvel, Shatmuli*
Oriya	:	*Sotabori*
Sanskrit	:	*Abhiru, Satavari*
Tamil	:	*Kilavari, Sadamoolam, Satavali, Thanirvitan*
Telugu	:	*Challagadde, Sadavari, Pilli-Gaddalu.*

Family	:	Liliaceae.
Appearance	:	The short, horizontal rootstock has long, thick roots and sends up young shoots, used as a vegetable. What look like leaves on the stem and branches are actually the filiform branches which are clustered in the axis of the scaly inconspicuous leaves. Flowers, greenish-white. Fruit, a red berry containing black seeds.
Distribution	:	Perennial plant, generally cultivated for food; may be found wild around gardens and wastelands. Found throughout tropical and subtropical India.
Medicinal Parts	:	Root, young shoots, seeds.

In Tradition

AILMENT	PRESCRIPTION
Body heat, fever, gonorrhoea, TB	: Powder the dried roots and store. Take 1 tsp twice a day with warm water.
Boils	: Steam the leaf gently. Spread a little ghee on its surface and tie over the area of boils.
Cough, nausea, noise in stomach, swelling in the throat, throat irritation	: Grind 1 tbsp seeds into a fine powder. Add 4 tbsp honey. Take 1 tsp thrice in daily.
Gout, lumbago, rheumatism	: Powder equal quantities of shatavari seeds, black cumin, fenugreek seeds and ajwain. Take 1 tsp every morning.
Indigestion, loss of taste	: Clean and boil 1 tbsp root in a cup of milk. Strain and add a little honey to improve the taste. Drink.
Leucorrhoea	: Mix 1 tsp leaf juice in a glass of milk and drink.
Mumps	: Grind shatavari and fenugreek seeds together in equal quantities in sufficient water into a fine paste. Apply on the affected areas.
Sexual debility	: Mix 1 tbsp root juice with 1 tbsp white butter and 1 teacup milk. Boil well. Add a little sugar, honey and long pepper. Drink for a few days.

Note: Individual results may vary.

A Word of Caution

Use of shatavari is not recommended when the kidneys are inflamed.

In Science

Chopra, R. N. et al. 1956. *Glossary of Indian Medicinal Plants.* New Delhi: Council of Scientific and Industrial Research. 28. (The plant's role in curing diarrhoea, dysentery; facilitating the secretion of milk and urine.)

Dange, P. S. et al. 1969. Amylase and lipase activities in the root of *Asparagus racemosus. Planta Medica* 17(4):393–395. (Root extract is enzyme-like.)

Dhankar, S. A. et al. 1986. Protective effect of *Asparagus racemosus* against induced abdominable sepsis. *Indian Drugs* 24(3):125–128. (The efficacy of shatavari against abdominal infection.)

Dhar, M. L. et al. 1968. Screening of Indian plants for biological activity. Part I. *Indian J. Exptl. Biol. 6:232.* (Anti-cancer, anti-amoebic, anti-viral and hypoglycaemic effects noted.)

Gaitonde, B. B. and M. Jetmalani. 1969. Antioxytocic and anti-ADH activity of saponin fraction isolated from *Asparagus racemosus* Willd. *Indian J. Pharm.* 31:175.

————. 1969. Antioxytocic action of saponin isolated from *Asparagus racemosus* Willd. (*Satavari*) on uterine muscle. *Arch. Int. Pharmacodyn.* 179:121.

Jetmalani, M. and B. B. Gaitonde. 1966. Pharmacology of *Asparagus racemosus (Satavari). Indian J. Pharm.* 28(12):341. No. 35.

————. 1966. Pharmacology of *Asparagus racemosus (Satavari). Indian J. Pharm.* 28(12):341. No. 36. (Evidence of action on mammary secretion in rats.)

————. 1967. A study on the pharmacology of various extracts of

Satavari (Asparagus racemosus Willd.). *J. Res. Indian Med.* 2:1. (Evidence of increased milk output.)

Karnick, C. R. 1972. Some aspects of crude Indian drug plants used in Ayurvedic system for *Madhumaya* (Diabetes). *Acta Phytother. Amst.* 19(8):141–149. (Evidence of the plant's anti-diabetic properties.)

Karnick, C. R. and S. N. Joshi. 1986. Studies on standardisation of ayurvedic crude drugs. Series 1- *Asparagus racemosus* Willd. (*Satavari*). *Nagarjun* 30(1):21–22.

Kishore, P. et al. 1980. Treatment of duodenal ulcer with *Asparagus racemosus* L. *J. Res. Ayur. Siddha* 1(3):409–416.

Landage, A. B. and J. L. Bose. 1970. Structure of disaccharide from *Asparagus racemosus (Shatamuli). Indian J. Chem.* 8:588.

Nanal, B. D. et al. 1974. Clinical study of *Satavari (Asparagus racemosus) J. Res. Indian Med.* 9(3):23–29. (Powdered root stops diarrhoea; shows gastric sedative action.)

Pande, T. N. and S. S. Rajagopalan. 1994. Comparative study of the regimen containing *Satavari* on *Amlapitta* (Acid Dyspepsia with or without ulcer). *J. Res. Ayur. Sid.* XV, 1&2: 23–34. (Shatavari mitigates discomfort caused by dyspepsia.)

Patel, A. B. and U. K. Kanitkar. 1969. *Asparagus racemosus* Willd. from Bordi as a galactagogue in buffaloes. *Indian Vet. J.* 46:718. (Good news for dairy-owners: milk-yield increases in buffaloes.)

Roy, R. N. et al. 1967. Preliminary pharmacological studies on different extracts of root of *Asparagus racemosus (Satawari)* Willd. *Indian J. Pharm.* 30:289. (Root extracts fight harmful amoebia, strengthen the heart and reduce blood pressure.)

———. 1971. Preliminary studies of extracts of root of *Asparagus racemosus (Shatawari)* Willd. (N. O. Liliaceae). *J. Res. Indian Med.* 6:132. (The root extract causes an increase in bleeding time in rabbits.)

Sabnis, P. B. et al. 1968. Effect of alcoholic extract of *Asparagus racemosus* on mammary glands of rats. *Indian J. Exptl. Biol.* 6:55. (Increase in milk secretion observed.)

Shimoyada, M. 1990. Antifungal activity of the saponin fraction obtained from *Asparagus officinalis* L. and its active principle. *Agri. Bio. Chem.* 54(10):2553–2557. (The plant's role as a destroyer of fungus.)

Singh, K. P. and R. H. Singh. 1986. Clinical trial of *satavari (Asparagus racemosus)* in duodenal ulcer. *J. Res. Ayur. Sid.* VII, 3&4:91–100. (Yet another weapon against ulcer.)

Singh, S. P. and C. D. Sharma. 1971. Less popular but an important vegetable, the *Asparagus. Indian Farmer's Digest* 4(1):17–18. (Importance of shatavari.)

Tennekoon, K. H. 1990. Evaluation of the galactologuic activity of *Asparagus falcatus. Ceylon J. Med. Sci.* 30(2):63–67.

10

Brahmi

Bacopa monnieri

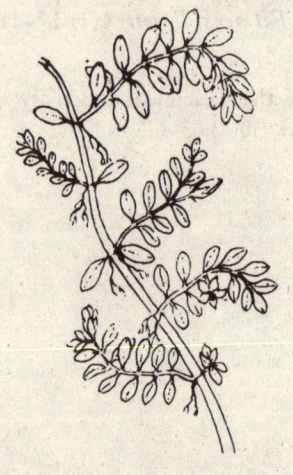

*Brahmi cures leprosy,
syphilis . . .*

—Bhava Prakasam

Brahmi and the Brain

The name brahmi often causes considerable confusion in the trade. Sometimes, mandukaparni (*Centella asiatica*) is also referred to as brahmi. Brahmi however refers solely to *Bacopa monnieri*. Like mandukaparni, brahmi is also credited with fine-tuning the mental faculies. Ayurveda has acknowledged the nourishing effect of brahmi on the human brain.

The plant contains an alkaloid, related to strychnine, but less toxic and hence capable of safe use by those who want to stimulate the intellect and the faculty of speech.

The drug is traditionally prescribed for nervous disorders such as insanity, epilepsy, neurasthenia, nervous breakdown, etc. A preliminary experiment conducted on rats reveals that the crude extract of this plant can improve their learning processes, as evidenced by better acquisition, improved retention and delayed extinction of information (Singh et al, 1978 and 1982). More recently, similar results have been obtained with Bacosides A and B isolated from this plant (Rastogi and Dhawan, 1982).

Alcoholic extracts of this plant have a tranquillizing effect on experimental animals. Bramhine, the alkaloid extracted from this plant, is reported to strengthen and tone the heart muscles.

In the Chinese System

Chinese doctors prescribe this plant for several ailments: backache, impotence, irregularity of the menstrual cycle, premature ejaculation, uterine problems, rheumatism, etc.

Profile

Botanical Names	:	*Bacopa monnieri* (L) Penn.
		Herpestis monnieria (L) H. B. K.
		Monnieri cuneifolia Mich.
		Lysimachia monnieri L.
English Name	:	Thyme-Leaved Gratiola.
Indian Names	:	Gujarati : *Jalbrahmi, Jalnevri*
		Hindi : *Barami, Brahmi, Jala Brahmi, Jal Neem, Safed Chamni*
		Kannada : *Nirbrahmi*
		Malayalam : *Barna, Nirbrahmi*
		Marathi : *Ghola*
		Sanskrit : *Brahmi, Sarasvati, Saumyalata*

69

	Tamil	: *Nirpirami, Piramiya-Poondu.*
	Telugu	: *Sambranichettu*
	Ayurvedic	: *Brahmi*
	Unani	: *Brahmi-Buti.*
Family	:	Scrophulariaceae.
Appearance	:	A small, prostrate herb with ascending branches. Roots arise on the nodes of the stem. Leaves, fleshy, oblong with obscure veins. Flowers, bluish-white or lilac. Fruit, egg-like with persistent style.
Distribution	:	Grows wild in the Indian plains, particularly in damp, moist surroundings.
Medicinal Parts	:	Leaves, the whole plant. *Dose:* 1 to 1^1/$_2$ tsp powder along with 1 tsp honey or 1 cup milk twice a day. 1 to 1^1/$_2$ tsp fresh juice twice a day.
Ayurvedic Preparations	:	*Brahmi Ghrita, Brahmi Oil.*
Unani Preparations	:	As a brain-tonic: *Ma'jun Brahmi.*

In Tradition

AILMENT	PRESCRIPTION
❦ Bronchitis, constipation, dyspepsia, fatigue, fevers, flatulence, insanity, nervous disorders, sterility	: Boil 1 teacup fresh juice of the plant along with 1 teacup ghee. Take 1 tsp twice a day for a few days. (*Note*: The relief is due to vomiting and purging brought about by the drug.)
❦ Cough in children	: Boil the crushed plant (about 2 cups),

make a poultice and place on the chest for half an hour. Repeat.

❧ Neuralgia, rheumatism, swellings

: Extract $1/2$ teacup leaf juice and mix with 1 teacup molten petroleum jelly. Apply when bearably warm. (*Note*: After each application, when the jelly has hardened, it can be re-melted and used repeatedly, say upto 1 month.)

❧ Rheumatism

: Extract the leaf juice and mix with hot paraffin and apply on the affected areas.

Note: Individual results may vary.

In Science

Aithal, H. N. and M. Sirsi. 1961. Pharmacological investigation of *Herpestis monnieri*. *Indian J.Pharm.* 23:2. (Tranquillizing effect on albino rats.)

Basu, N. et al. 1967. Chemical examination of *Bacopa monnieri* Wettst. III- Bacoside B. *Indian J.Chem.* 5:85–86. (Active principles isolated.)

Chandel, R. S. et al. 1977. Bacogenin A: A new sapogenin from *Bacopa monnieri*. *Phytochemistry* 16:141–143.

Chatterjee, N. et al. 1963. Chemical examination of *Bacopa monnieri* Wettst. Part I: Isolation of chemical constituents. *Indian J.Chem.* 1:212–215. (Chemical constituents described.)

———. 1965. Chemical examination of *Bacopa monnieri* Wettst. Part II: The constitution of Bacoside A. *Indian J.Chem.* 3:24–29. (The plant's role improving the memory studied.)

Kulshreshtha, D. K. and R. P. Rastogi. 1975. Absolute structures of the novel genins, bacogenin A and A2 from bacoside isolated from *Bacopa monnieri*. *Indian J.Chem.* 13:309–313.

Malhotra C. L. and P. K. Das. 1959. Pharmacological studies of *Herpestis monnieri* Linn. (*Brahmi*). *Indian J. Med. Res.* 47:294.

Rastogi, R. P and M. L. Dhar. 1960. Chemical examination of *Bacopa monnieri* Wettst. *J. Sci. Industr. Res.* 19B:455–456. (Chemical composition.)

Sharma, R. et al. 1987. Efficacy of *Bacopa monnieri* in revitalising intellectual functions in children. *Jour. Res. Edn. Ind. Med.* 6(1-2):1–10. (Revitalizes the intellect.)

Singh, H. K. and B. N. Dhawan. 1978. Effect of *Bacopa monnieri* on the learning ability of rats. *Indian J. Pharmacol.* 10:72. (Facilitates the learning process.)

———. 1982. Effect of *Bacopa monnieri* (Brahmi) extract on avoidance responses in rats. *J. Ethnopharmacol.* 5:205–214. (The plant's impact on the brain and the mental responses studied.)

Singh, R. H. et al. 1979. Studies on the anti-anxiety effect of the *medhya rasayana* drug *brahmi (Bacopa monnieri* L.) Part II. Experimental Studies. *J. Res. Ind. Med. Yoga. & Homoeop.* 14(3-4):1–6. (The plant plays a role in eliminating anxiety.)

11

Indian Barberry

Berberis aristata

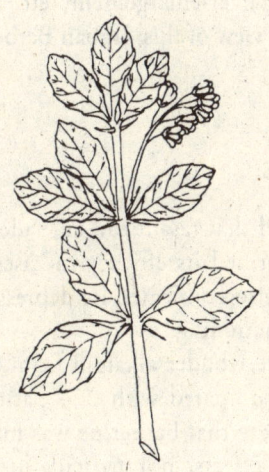

Dharu Haridra, one of the ten drugs that reduce corpulence.

—Charaka Samhita

The Uses of Rasaut

By boiling the roots, root bark and lower portions of the stems of this plant and on straining the liquid, a filtrate is obtained. The solution is evaporated and the resultant semi-solid mass is known to folk-medicine as rasaut.

Rasaut is used as a local application in afflictions of the eyelids; it is painted over the eyelids in the case of chronic ophthalmia. The Kurumbas, a tribal community in the Nedugalcombay in the Nilgiris use the root-paste for the treatment of stomach ache. A number of scientific experiments and clinical trials conducted recently have confirmed the relevance of rasaut in treating stomach problems.

Rasaut and Turmeric

Interestingly, one finds almost identical properties in both rasaut and turmeric. Both are useful in the treatment of jaundice. Several ailments such as colitis, dysentery, liver-enlargement, etc. can also be treated effectively by both. In view of this, Indian Barberry is also known as Wood Tumeric.

Experimental Conclusions

Experimental studies have confirmed that rasaut can cure ulcers. Clinical trials on rabbits have confirmed its efficacy in cases of acute diarrhoea. Experiments have also confirmed its depressant action on respiration and heart functioning.

Clinical trials with berberine, the wonder alkaloid from this plant, in 356 patients of cholera, compared with 264 patients treated with chloramphenicol, indicate that berberine was much more effective. It showed no side effects, nor toxicity in the doses tried (Lahiri and Dutta, 1967).

Based on recent experiments, the following conclusions have been reached on the efficacy of berberine:
- Berberine acts in severe diarrhoea and cholera by reducing the increase of capillary permeability.
- It exercises effective control over gastroenteritis.
- It exhibits anti-inflammatory action on acute, sub-acute and chronic models of inflammation.
- Berberine acts directly on blood vessels to produce a hypotensive effect.
- It stimulates the heart and increases the rate and amplitude of respiration.

- It reduces rectal temperature.
- Berberine possesses anticholinesterase-like and local anaesthetic action.
- It prevents the death of young rabbits suffering from cholera, if administered early.

According to scientists of the All India Institute of Medical Sciences, New Delhi, berberine 'may prove a practical remedy for large-scale use in trachoma patients' (Sabir and Bhide, 1971).

Profile

Botanical Name	: *Berberis aristata* D.C.	
English Name	: Indian Barberry.	
Indian Names	: Bengali	: *Darhaldi, Daruhaldi*
	Hindi	: *Dar-Hald, Daru-Haldi, Kilmora, Kingora, Rasaut*
	Kashmiri	: *Rasvat*
	Malayalam	: *Maradarisina*
	Marathi	: *Daru-Hald*
	Punjabi	: *Kashmal*
	Sanskrit	: *Daru Haridra*
	Tamil	: *Maramanjal*
	Ayurvedic	: *Dhaaruharidra*.
Family	: Berberidaceae.	
Appearance	: A spiny shrub; bark, pale yellowish-brown, deeply furrowed; branches, shining reddish-brown; leaves, glossy dark-green above and glossy pale-green beneath; flowers, golden yellow in drooping clusters; berries, spindle-shaped, bluish-purple. Seeds few.	
Distribution	: Grows in the temperate Himalayas from	

the Indus eastwards to Bhutan, Kulu and Kumaon, and the Nilgiris at an altitude of 1800–3500 m.

Medicinal Parts : Root bark, stem.

Other Related Species : *Berberis asiatica* Roxb.
Berberis lycium Royle.
Berberis vulgaris (English Names: European Barberry, Jaundice Berry, Pepperidge).

In Tradition

AILMENT   PRESCRIPTION

↓ Bleeding piles : Dilute rasaut in water (1:30). Use the solution to wash the affected areas. Mix 1/8 tsp powdered rasaut in 1 tsp butter and take.

↓ Boils, pimples : Mix 1 tsp butter and 1/4 tsp camphor with 1 tsp powdered rasaut and make a fine paste. Apply on the affected parts frequently.

↓ Constipation, fevers, ulcers : Mix 1/8 tsp rasaut in 1 teacup hot water and drink. (*Caution:* The root bark is laxative.)

↓ Eye diseases, ophthalmia : Apply rasaut externally over the eyelids.

↓ Mouth-ulcer : Grind together equal quantities of the dried leaves of the following plants: Indian barberry, jasmine, liquorice and chebulic myrobalan. Sieve well to collect a very fine powder. Bottle and store. At the time of application add 1 tsp honey to 1 tsp mixture and make a smooth paste. Apply all over the interior of the mouth.

❦ Jaundice : Mix 1 tsp honey in 1 cup decoction of rasaut and drink.

❦ Painful urination : Mix $1/2$ tsp amla powder in 1 cup decoction of rasaut. Add 1 tsp honey and drink.

❦ Ulcers : Wash the wounds frequently with a decoction of rasaut.

Note: Individual results may vary.

A Word of Caution

Berberine in excess can cause pronounced or even fatal poisoning.

In Science

Akhter, M. H. et al. 1977. Anti-inflammatory effect of berberine in rats injected locally with cholera toxin. *Indian J. Med. Res.* 65(1):133–141. (Anti-inflammatory properties.)

Bhatnagar, S. S. et al. 1961. Biological activity of Indian Medicinal Plants Part I. Antibacterial, anti-tubercular and anti-viral action. *Indian J. Med. Res.* 49(5):799–813. (Antibacterial action confirmed.)

Bhide, M. B. et al. 1969. Absorption, distribution and excretion of berberine. *Indian J. Med. Res.* 57:2128. (Fights severe diarrhoea and cholera.)

Central Council for Research in Indian Medicine and Homoeopathy. 1978. *Tribal Pockets of Nilgiris—Recordings of the Field Study on Medicinal Flora and Health Practices*. New Delhi.

Chakravarti, K. K. et al. 1950. Alkaloidal constituents of the bark of *Berberis aristata* (Rassaut). *J. Sci. Industr. Res*. 9B:142.

Chopra, R. N. et al. 1956. *Glossary of Indian Medicinal Plants*. New Delhi: Council of Scientific and Industrial Research. 36. (Fights skin diseases.)

Choudhury, V. P. et al. 1972. Berberine in giardiasis. *Indian Pediatrics* 9:143. (Anti-protozoal action confirmed.)

Dhar M. L. et al. 1968. Screening of Indian plants for biologial activity. Part I. *Indian J. Exptl. Biol*. 6:232. (CNS depressant, anti-cancer properties.)

Dutta, N. K. and M. V. Pendse. 1962. Usefulness of berberine (an alkaloid from *Berberis aristata*) in the treatment of cholera (experimental). *Indian J. Med. Res*. 50(5):1732–1736.

Dutta, N. K. and N. S. Iyer. Anti-amoebic value of berberine and Kurchi alkaloids. *J. Indian Med. Assn*. 50:349. (Anti-protozoal activity.)

Ghosh A. K. et al. 1983. Effect of Berberine chloride on *Leishmania donovani*. *Indian J. Med. Res*. 78:407–416.

Godbole, S. H. and G. S. Pendse. 1960. Antibacterial properties of some plants. *Indian J. Pharm*. 22(2):39.

Halder, R. K. et al. 1970. Pharmacological investigations on Berberine hydrochloride. *Indian J. Pharmac*. 2:26. (Anti-inflammatory properties studied.)

Imam, Z. 1977. Ancient medicine in eye diseases. *Sci. Rep*. 14(6):393. (Antitrachoma efficacy.)

Javed, A. et al. 1985. Zakaria al-Razi's treatise on botanical, animal and mineral drugs for cancer. *Hamdard* 28(3):76–99.

Lahiri, S. C and N. K. Dutta. 1967. Berberine and chloramphenicol in the treatment of cholera and severe diarrhoea. *J.Indian Med. Assn*.

48:1. (Antibacterial properties: berberine out-performs chloramphenicol.)

Mahl, B. S. and V. P. Trivedi. 1972. Vegetable anti-fertility drugs of India. *Quart. J. Crude Drug Res.* 12(3):1922–1928.

Rahman, A. and A. A. Ansari. 1983. Alkaloids of *Berberis aristata*— isolation of aromoline and oxyber berine. *J. Chem. Soc. Pakistan.* 5:283.

Sabir, M. 1969. Some pharmacological studies of berberine, an alkaloid which occurs in *Berberis aristata* and other plants. *M. D. Thesis.* New Delhi: All India Institute of Medical Sciences. (Local anaesthetic and CNS-depressant activity.)

Sabir, M. et al. 1976. Experimental study of the antitrachoma action of berberine. *Indian J. Med. Res.* 64(8):1160–1167. (The ancient Ayurvedic claims of the role of the plant in eye diseases upheld.)

Sabir, M. and N. K. Bhide. 1971. Study of some pharmacological actions of Berberine. *Indian J. Physiol Pharmacol.* 15:117. (Study conducted on mice.)

———. 1971. *In vitro* antiheparin action of berberine on the dog and human blood. *Indian J. Physiol. Pharmacol.* 15:97. ('Berberine may prove a practical remedy for large-scale use in trachoma patients.')

Sharda, D. C. 1970. Berberine in treatment of diarrhoea in infancy and childhood. *J. Indian Med. Assn.* 54(1):22–24. (Gastroentritis in children controlled.)

Singh, R. H. 1978. Critical analysis of the studies done on indigenous, anti-inflammatory and anti-arthritic drugs during post-independent era. *Rheumatism* 99–108. (Anti-inflammatory properties.)

Verma, R. L. 1933. Berberine sulphate in chronic trachoma. *Indian Med. Gaz.* 68:122. (Clinical report.)

Vohora, S. B. 1985. What is purification of blood? *Hamdard* 28(1):72–84. (Useful in skin diseases.)

12

Flame of the Forest

Butea monosperma

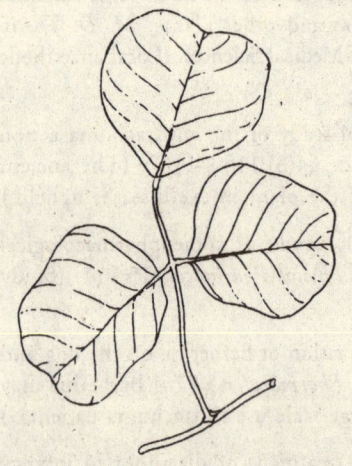

*Red petals of kimsuka, the
nail marks from the
passionate embraces of the
Lady Spring . . .*

—Kalidasa,
Kumarasambhavam (1st
Century A.D.)

Tree of Myriad Metaphors

The beautiful flowers of this tree when in full bloom give the
impression that the entire forest has been set afire and hence the
popular name Flame of the Forest. Kalidasa was particularly
fond of describing the beauty of this tree: the jungle resembles
to him a blaze of fire, the forest-floor, like a coy bride wrapped
in red garments. The flowers also bring to mind the beak of a
parrot and hence the Sanskrit name, *Kimsuka* ('like a parrot'.)

The tree finds frequent mention in the Vedas. Believed to be
a tree from the Heavens, it is an obvious choice for many religious

rites of the Hindus. In Buddhist mythology, Queen Mahamaya is reported to have grasped a branch of this tree at the moment of the birth of Siddhartha, who later became the Buddha.

Flowers

The flowers are not only beautiful but also functional: helpful in alleviating morbid *pitta* and *kapha*, they reduce excessive thirst, burning sensations, and pain caused during micturition. The flowers also cure several skin ailments.

Apart from the flowers, the bark, gum, leaves, and seeds all find their application in ethno-medical practices.

Bark

The bark is found to be useful in treating abdominal tumours, colic, intestinal worms, bleeding piles, ulcers, haemorrhages, amenorrhoea and dysmenorrhoea.

Gum

The red-coloured gum known as Bengal Kino obtained from the tree is also referred to as Kamarkas as it is extensively used by women in cases of backache. Its tannin content renders it useful in treating diarrhoea and dysentery. It is also reported to be useful in cases of haemorrhage in the stomach and bladder, and is in addition a well-known astringent.

Seeds

The seeds are a well-known anthelmintic agent. The majority of preparations from the flame of the forest are used to fight worm-infestation. Some laboratory studies have confirmed the usefulness of seeds in eliminating roundworm infection.

Profile

Botanical Names	:	*Butea monosperma* (Lam.) Taub. *Butea frondosa* Koen ex Roxb.	
English Names	:	Bengal Kino, Flame of the Forest, Bastard Teak, Parrot Tree.	
Indian Names	:	Bengali	: *Kinaka, Palas, Polashi*
		Gujarati	: *Khakria, Khakro*
		Hindi	: *Chalcha, Dhak, Palasa, Tesu*
		Kannada	: *Muttagamara*
		Malayalam	: *Brahmavriksham, Chamata, Kimshukam, Mukkalappuyam, Muriku, Plasu, Shamata*
		Marathi	: *Kakracha, Palas, Paras*
		Oriya	: *Kinjuko, Polaso*
		Sanskrit	: *Kimsuka*
		Tamil	: *Chamata, Kali, Katumurukku, Palaasu, Kinjugam, Kiruminasanam Kirumisatturu, Vaadhabodham, Porasu*
		Telugu	: *Kimsukamu, Moduga, Modugu, Palasamu*
		Urdu	: *Palash Papra*
		Ajmer, Rajasthan	: *Chaura.*
Family	:	Fabaceae.	
Sub-family	:	Faboideae.	

Appearance	:	A tree with grey/light brown bark. It is often the host of the lac insect. Leaves, 3-lobed with stalk. Flowers deep orange/red, in clusters. Calyx with velvet-like silky hairs. Pod, stalked with a single seed. The tree shows untidy growth, with a twisted and gnarled trunk.
Distribution	:	All over India upto 1000m. Occcurs naturally in deciduous forests. Also in the tropical Himalayas, Sri Lanka, Malaysia and South East Asia.
Medicinal Parts	:	Leaf, flower, seed, bark, gum.
Ayurvedic Preparations	:	*Palasa-Beejadi-Churna, Krimihara-Churna, Krimighatini-Bati, Palasa-Beejadi-Kshara* etc.
Unani Preparations	:	*Ma'jun Zangbil, Ma'jun Supari Pak* (to cure leucorrhoea).

In Tradition

AILMENT	PRESCRIPTION
✤ Boils	: Apply a paste of the leaves on the affected parts.
	: Steam a handful of flowers and bandage the boils with these.
✤ Cough, dropsy, heaviness in head	: Add a piece of bark to boiling water and use to drink from frequently, in place of water.
✤ Dhobi's itch	: Grind 1 tsp seeds with 1 tsp lime juice

and apply the paste on the affected parts.

♦ Dysentery : Take 1/4 tsp finely ground powder of the gum and 1/4 tsp powdered cinnamon with some warm water.

♦ Excessive thirst : Crush the bark into small, tiny pieces. Soak in water and mix with sugar candy. Chew 1/2 tsp.

♦ Intestinal disorders : Soak the seeds for 4–5 hours. Remove the seed-coat and dry the kernel. Powder and store. *Dose:* Mix 1/2 tsp of the powder in 1 tsp honey. Take thrice a day for 3 days. On the fourth day (morning), take 1 tbsp castor oil with 1 cup milk to purge the parasites from the digestive tract.

♦ Ringworm : Crush 1 tbsp seeds and dust on the affected areas.

♦ Snakebite : To remove the poison due to snakebite in some forest areas of South India, a mixture of equal quantities of the bark of palash and ginger are ground together in water and administered.

♦ Stomach upset : Soak a handful of leaves in a pot of water and drink frequently.

♦ Swelling of testicles : Crush and boil the flowers and bandage them over the scrotum.

♦ Throat ulceration : Dissolve the gum in a little water and apply with a cotton swab on the throat.

❖ Urine retention : Use *Butea* leaves to foment the pubic region.

: Boil a fistful of flowers in 1 litre water. Strain and drink frequently with a little rock-salt.

Note: Individual results may vary.

A Word of Caution

Prolonged oral administration for 2 months produced marked toxicity in the kidneys and anaemia in rats, dogs and rabbits. Congestion in the liver, spleen and lungs was also observed. The stomach showed gross dilation and chronic inflammation (Sachdeva, K. S. et al, 1961). Prolonged and unnecessary use of this drug can result in undesirable side effects.

In Science

Bhatnagar, S. S. et al. 1961. Biological activities of Indian medicinal plants. Part I. Antibacterial, anti-tubercular and antifungal action. *Indian J. Med. Res.* 49(5):799–813. (Stops fungal growth.)

Chakraborty, B. 1977. Pharmacological investigation with *Butea monosperma*. *Sci. and Cult.* 43(8):344–345. (Causes excitability, hurried respiration and tremors in mice.)

Chaudhary, R. R. et al. 1980. Review of plants screened for anti-fertility activity. *Bull. Medico-Ethno-Bot. Res.* 1(3):420–427. (Seed-extract shows considerable anti-fertility activity.)

Chopra, R. N. et al. 1956. *Glossary of Indian Medicinal Plants*. New Delhi: Council of Scientific and Industrial Resarch. 42. (Aphrodisiac properties noted.)

Dhar, M. L. et al. 1968. Screening of Indian plants for biological activity. Part V. *Indian J. Exptl. Biol.* 6(4):232–247. (Relieves spasms.)

———. 1973. Screening of Indian plants for biological activity. *Indian J. Exptl. Biol.* 11(1):43–54. (Facilitates urine flow.)

Garg, S. K. 1970. Anti-fertility screening of plants. *Indian J. Med. Res.* 58(9):1285–1289.

———. 1971. Chemical examination of the seed oil of *Butea parviflora*. *Fette Seif. Anstrichm* 73:473.

Garg, S. K. et al. 1969. Investigation on *Butea monosperma* (Lam.) Kuntze. *Indian J. Med. Res.* 57:1946. (No significant anti-implantation activity in albino rats.)

———. 1978. Screening of Indian plants for anti-fertility activity. *Indian J. Exptl. Biol.* 16:1077.

Gupta, S. R. et al. 1970. The glucosides of *Butea monosperma*. *Phytochemistry* 9:2231.

Hasan et al. 1982. Review of scientific studies on anthelmintic fruit plants. *J. Sci. Res. Pl. Med.* 3(1):6–12. (Destroys worms.)

Hashmi, S. and A. M. Khan. 1990. Pharmacognosy of *plaspapra (Butea monosperma* Kuntze): An anthelmintic drug of Unani medicine. *Indian J. Unani Med.* 1(1):55–60.

Jawaharlal, et al. 1976. *In vitro* anthelmintic action of some indigenous medicinal plants on *Acarida galli* worms. *Indian J. Physiol. Pharmacol.* 20(2):64–68. (More effective than piperazine in fighting vigorously mobile worms.)

Kapila, K. et al. 1970. Anti-fertility effect on alcoholic extract and its crystalline fraction obtained from *Butea frondosa* petals. *J. Indian Med. Asoc.* 55:60. (No significant anti-fertility role.)

Kalysa, B. R. and P. A. Kurup. 1968. Anthelmintic activity, toxicity and other pharmacological properties of palasonin, the active principle of *Butea frondosa* seeds and its piperazine salt. *Indian J. Med. Res.* 56:1818. (Worm-destroying properties compared favourably with piperazine and santonin.)

Khanna, U. 1966. Effect of *Butea monosperma* on the fertility of female rats. *Indian J. Pharm.* 28(12):343. (Hot alcoholic extract exhibits anti-fertility effect.)

Khanna, U. et al. 1980. Investigation on *Butea monosperma* (Lam.) Kuntze. *Indian J. Pharm.* 56:1575. (Alcoholic seed-extract inhibits ovulation in mice.)

Kholkute, S. D. 1976. Screening of Indian medicinal plants for anti-fertility potentiality. *Planta Med.* 29(2):151–155.

Laumas, K. R. and J. P. Uniyal. 1966. A preliminary report on the anti-estrogenic activity of the petals of *Butea frondosa* flower. *Indian J. Exp. Biol.* 4:246.

Masilamani, G. et al. 1981. Study on Karappan (Eczema). *J. Res. Ayur. Siddha* 2(2):109–121. (The seed powder taken internally and also dusted externally causes significant improvement in eczema.)

Murti, P. B. R. and T. R. Seshadri. 1940. Occurence of free butein and butrin in the flowers of *Butea frondosa*. *Proc. Indian. Acad. Sci.* 12A:477.

Nazimuddin, S. K. et al. 1990. Protective effect of *Gul-e-tesu (Butea monosperma* (Lam.) Kuntze) flowers in experimental liver-injury. *Indian J. Unani Med.* 1(1):1–8. (Protects the liver from injuries.)

Rane, A. and N. D. Grampurohit. 1998. Hepatoprotective activity of *Pterocarpus marsupium* Roxb. and *Butea frondosa* Koen. ex. Roxb. *Indian J. Pharmaceutical Sci.* 60(3):182–184. (The extracts showed definite liver-protective activity.)

Rao, P. S. and T. R. Seshadri. 1941. Constitution of butrin. *Proc. Indian Acad. Sci.* 14A:29.

Razdan, M. K. et al. 1969. Anti-fertility effect and some pharmacological actions of *Butea frondosa* seed extracts. *Indian J. Physiol. Pharmacol.* 13:239.

————. 1970. Study of the anti-estrogenic activity of alcoholic extracts of petals and seeds of *Butea frondosa*. *Indian J. Physiol. Pharmacol.* 14:37.

Sachdeva, K. S. et al. 1965. Toxicity of *Butea frondosa*. *Indian J. Pharm.* 27(3):96.

———. 1965. Toxicity of *Butea frondosa*. *Indian J. Pharm.* 27:253.

Seshadri, T. R. and R. K. Trikha. 1971. Proanthocyanidins from the bark and gum of *Butea monosperma*. *Indian J. Chem.* 9:1201.

Shah, K. G. et al. 1992. Phyto-chemical studies and anti-oestrogenic activity of *Butea frondosa* flowers. *Indian J. Pharmac. Sci.* 52(6):272–275.

Shaw, B. P. and A. K. Tripathi. 1982. Clinical assessment of *Palas-beej* (seeds of *Butea monosperma)* on *Ascaris lumbsicoides*. *Nagarjun* 26(3):53–56. (Positive action recorded.)

Shome, U. et al. 1979. Pharmacognostic studies on the flower of *Butea monosperma* (Lam.) Kuntze. *Indian J. Pharm. Sci.* 41(5):253. (Medicinal use of the flowers verified.)

Siddiqui, H. H. and M. C. Inamdar. 1964. Preliminary pharmacological examination of *Butea superba* seeds. *Indian J. Pharm.* 25:270. (Seed oil reduces blood pressure.)

Sukh Dev, 1983. Natural products in medicine–present status and future prospects. *Curr. Sci.* 52(20):947–956. (Cures worm-infestation.)

Tandon, S. P. et al. 1969. Chemical examination of the root of *Butea monosperma*. *Proc. Nat. Acad. Sci. India.* A, 32:237.

Zafar, R. et al. 1991. Anti-microbial and preliminary phyto-chemical studies on leaves of *Butea monosperma*. *Indian J. Forestry* 12(4):328–329.

13

Arkh

Calotropis gigantea

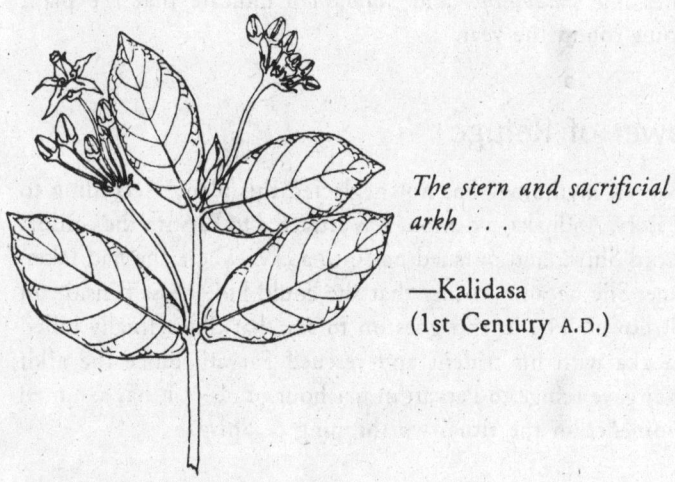

The stern and sacrificial
arkh . . .

—Kalidasa
(1st Century A.D.)

Attractive Commoner

Typical Indian common lands, though ostensibly given over to
rank wild growth and unwanted beasts of burden like donkeys,
have long been barely recognized sources of community well-
being. Donkeys and arkh, both inseparable from the common
lands, seem to share a similar destiny: both, though useful, are
not cared for and left to fend for themselves in the wilderness.

There are two varieties of arkh: one with white flowers and
the other with light blue flowers. The flowers, although handsome
and prominent-looking, have somehow been neglected by poets
and painters alike.

Although the plant is attractive to look at and medicinally useful, it gives off a foul smell. And there perhaps, lies the rub!

Ever-in-Bloom

The plant's Sanskrit names are descriptive: *arkah*, *vasukah*, *pratapah* and *vikiranah* refer to its strong, caustic action. Other names like *sadapushpa* and *sadasumah* indicate that the plant blooms round the year.

Flower of Refuge

However, mythology has not neglected this plant. According to one story, Andhaka, a demon, was attracted to Parvati, the consort of Lord Shiva, and pursued her into a cave where she had taken refuge. She became so tiny that she could hide herself inside an arkh flower. The legend goes on to say that Shiva finally killed Andhaka with his trident and rescued Parvati. Since the arkh flower gave refuge to Parvati in her hour of need, it has assumed prominence in the ritual worshipping of Shiva.

The Drug

Arkh which belongs to a group of purgatives, is hot, acrid and laxative. Experiments conducted in laboratories and clinical studies undertaken in recent years have pointed to the tremendous medicinal potential locked in this plant.

Leaves

The terminal leaves of arkh have proved their usefulness in the treatment of migraine. Fresh leaves are used by villagers foment swellings. Tinctures made from the leaves are administered to relieve asthma, cold, cough, digestive disorders and fevers.

In the Unani tradition, the milky leaf juice, which is purgative, is the main ingredient in medicinal preparations that treat bronchial congestions, eosinophilia and sexual debility. Incidentally, Vatsyayana who lived in the 4th century and who was the author of the famous treatise on love, the *Kama Sutra* refers to the aphrodisiac quality of arkh.

The Kurumbas, a tribal community in Mavinahalla in the Nilgiris use the leaf juice to facilitate the easy removal of thorns.

The Root

The root is used as an abortifacient, while the root bark is considered a substitute for ipecac in the treatment of dysentery and bronchial troubles. The ethanolic extract applied to patients suffering from cancerous ulcers showed a 60 degree growth regression.

Calotropin, extracted from the roots, has been found to be effective in fertility control as it inhibited the motility of sperm.

Several clinical trials conducted recently have confirmed the efficacy of the root bark in the control of diarrhoea and dysentery.

Profile

Botanical Names	:	*Calotropis gigantea* (Linn.) R. Br.
		Calotropis procera (Ait) R. Br.
English Name	:	Swallow Wort, Madar.
Indian Names	:	Bengali	: *Akanda*
		Hindi	: *Ak, Akada, Akond, Arkh, Madar*
		Kannada	: *Arka, Ekke*

91

Malayalam	: *Eriku, Eruku*
Sanskrit	: *Arkh, Arkah*
Tamil	: *Velleruku, Arkam, Eruku*
Telugu	: *Jilledu*
Urdu	: *Madar, Safed Ak.*

Family	:	Asclepiadaceae.
Appearance	:	Erect, pale greyish shrub covered with white cottony coat. Leaves, simple, ear-shaped at base. Flowers, lilac or dull white. Fruits are in pairs, somewhat resembling mangoes, containing loose, silky and fibrous growths.
Distribution	:	All over India, especially the wastelands.
Medicinal Parts	:	Flowers, latex, leaves, root.
Ayurvedic Preparations	:	*Ark Lavanam, Ark Tailam, Arkeshwara Wati.*
Unani Preparations	:	*Hab Seen, Kushta Qarnu-Eil, Kushta Shangraf.*

In Tradition

AILMENT	PRESCRIPTION
✤ Ascites, leprosy, leucoderma, ringworm, scorpion sting, skin diseases, tumours, ulcers	: Latex applied locally.
✤ Boils	: Take 2 tsp latex of the madar plant and mix thoroughly with powdered

turmeric and apply on the boils repeatedly.

❧ Boils, pimples : Add 1 tsp ajwain to 1 tbsp milky juice of the plant and leave overnight. In the morning, roast the soaked seeds over a low fire and grind them into a very fine powder. Now add a little yoghurt and apply over the affected areas.

❧ Breathing problems : Grind equal quantities of the flowers, cloves and black pepper. Take a pinch of the mixture with warm water. (*Caution:* Excess intake may cause vomiting or diarrhoea.)

❧ Bronchitis, cold, cough, fatigue, insect bite, leprosy : Take the required quantity of root bark and powder finely. Mix an equal quantity of palm sugar with it and store. Take one or two pinches mixed in a glass of warm milk at bedtime. (*Caution:* Excess intake may cause vomiting or diarrhoea.)

❧ Cholera (initial stages) : Powder the root bark and mix into it some ginger juice and add an equal quantity of black pepper. Roll into pea-sized pills. *Dose:* A pill every two hours along with 1/2 cup hot decoction of 1 cardamom and 1 tsp pudina for a few days.

❧ Cold, cough, epilepsy, headache : Take 1 porcelain cup of rice. Add 1 tsp latex. Allow it to dry under the sun for 7 days. Repeat with a similar addition of latex 3 times and re-dry. When totally dry, powder thoroughly, sieve and collect only the very fine powder. Mix with this 2 tsp finely ground camphor. Use as snuff. (*Note:* If fits of sneezing occur, wash the face well in running water.)

❧ Colic, gastralgia : Grind 1 tbsp flowers along with 1 tbsp ajwain, 2 tsp dried ginger and 1 tsp black salt. Add a little lime juice and roll into pea-sized pills. *Dose:* 1 pill with 1 cup hot water.

❧ Deafness : Warm a ripe yellow leaf and squeeze the juice in drops into the ears. Continue for a fortnight. (*Note:* This treatment may be beneficial only in certain types of deafness.)

❧ Dental caries : Rub the latex on the affected teeth.

❧ Earache,
ear diseases,
ear infection,
pus in ear
: Pluck some ripe yellowish leaves and express about 1/4 cup juice. Mix in the same amount of gingelly oil. Add 1/4 tsp each of the following powders: calamus, cinnamon and garlic. Add 2 tsp asafoetida powder. Boil the mixture over a low fire till it thickens. Filter through a cloth. When cool, use as ear drops.

❧ Enlargement of the
abdomen, painful
joints, swelling
: Lightly roasted leaves are applied locally.

❧ Gout : Crush 1 cup each of the leaves of

94

calotropis, dhatura, castor and
Common Milk Hedge (*Thoohar*) and
extract their juice. Add equal quantities
of gingelly oil and boil till all traces of
moisture have evaporated. Massage the
affected parts with this oil and bandage.

❧ Headache

: Warm the leaf over a flame and tie on
the forehead. (*Caution:* Avoid contact
of the milky juice of the leaves with
the eyes).

❧ Headache,
migraine

: Take $1/2$ litre gingelly oil and add to
this 2 tbsp calotropis flowers and 2 tsp
each turmeric powder, garlic paste and
black pepper powder. Boil the mixture
thoroughly over a low flame till the
solution thickens. Cool, filter and store
in a bottle. Take 2–3 tsp of this oil
and massage the scalp well. Wash after
little while. This may be done thrice a
week for better results.

❧ Leprosy wounds

: Take equal quantities of leaf and root
bark, and dry thoroughly. Grind to a
fine powder. Mix with coconut oil and
apply externally. (During this treatment,
it is advisable to eat only cooked rice
with milk or curd and without salt.)

❧ Mumps

: Tie the leaves over the affected areas.

❧ Swellings

: Extract the milky exudate from the
plant and apply repeatedly.

❧ Swelling in feet
and hands

: Blend together 1 cup each of the juices
of madar leaf, dhatura leaf and ginger.

Boil and allow to cool before applying on the affected parts.

❧ Swollen joints : Warm up gingelly oil and fry some leaves in it over a low flame and apply locally.

❧ Whitlow : Warm the leaf over a flame. Smear with a mixture of slaked lime and turmeric. Tie around the affected finger.

Note: Individual results may vary.

A Word of Caution

There are several poisonous substances in arkh e.g. Usheerin, Calotoxin, Calactin, etc. The plant should therefore be handled very carefully. Internal use may induce vomiting and may cause poisoning. It is advisable to wash the hands with soap and water immediately after handling any part of the plant. In case of any poisoning due to calotropis, gingelly oil (2 tsp) is to be taken 3 or 4 times a day. Yet another useful remedy for calatropis poisoning is a mixture of seasame seeds and jaggery, a sweetmeat commonly available in Indian households.

Leaf juice of tamarind or castor oil can also eliminate any traces of poisoning.

In Science

Anjaneyulu, V. and L. R. Row. 1968. The triterpene of *Calotropis gigantea*. *Curr. Sci.* 37:158. (Isolated from the root bark.)

Atal, C. K. and P. D. Sethi. 1962. Proteolytic activity of some Indian plants. III. Isolation, properties and kinetic studies of calotropain.

Planta Med. 10:77. (Calotropain, the enzyme is more active than its cousins papain, bromelin and ficin.)

Balakrishna, K. J. et al. 1945. Chemical composition of *Calotropis gigantea.* V. Further examination of the latex and root bark. *Proc. Indian Acad. Sci.* 22A:143.

Balakrishna, N. J. et al. 1945. Chemical composition of *Calotropis gigantea. Proc. Indian Acad. Sci.* 22A:138.

Basu, K. P. and M. C. Nath. 1934. Calosterol: A sterol present in the milky juice of *Calotropis gigantea. Biochem. J.* 28:156.

Bhakuni, D. S. et al. 1969. Screening of Indian plants for biological activity. Part II. *Indian J. Exp. Biol.* 7:250.

Bhatnagar, S. K. and S. K. Verma. 1986. Effects of 50% ethanol extract of *Calotropis procera* Ait. f. on ulcers caused by assorted types of carcinoma. *Jour Econ. Tax. Bot.* 8(2):489–490. (Useful against cancer.)

Bose, S. M. and W. M. Krishna. 1958. Purification and properties of the protease of latex of madar *(Calotropis gigantea). Enzymologia* 19:186; *Chem. Abstr.* 1959, 53:22270a.

Central Council for Research in Indian Medicine and Homoeopathy. 1978. *Tribal Pockets of Nilgiris—Recordings of the Field Study on Medicinal Flora and Health Practices.* New Delhi.

Chen, K. K. et al. 1942. The digitalis-like principle of Calotropis compounds with other cardiac substances. *J. Pharmac. Exp. Ther.* 74:223. (Helpful in cardiac diseases.)

Crout, D. H. G. and C. H. Hassall. 1963. Cardenolides. V. Constitution of Calactinic acid. *J. Chem. Soc.* 85.

————. 1964. Cardenolides. VI. Uscharidin, calotropin and calotoxin. *J. Chem. Soc.* 2187.

Derashri, H. R. and G. F. Shah. 1965. Preliminary pharmacological investigation of the roots of *Calotropis procera* R. Br. *Indian J. Pharm.* 27:278. (Medicine in the roots.)

Dhar, M. L. et al. 1968. Screening of Indian plants for biological activity. Part I. *Indian J. Exp. Biol.* 6:232.

Dhawan, B. N. and P. N. Saxena. 1968. Evaluation of some indigenous drugs for stimulating effect on the rat uterus. A preliminary report. *Indian J. Med. Res.* 46:808.

Garg, L. C. et al. 1963. Anthelmintic activity of calotropin and bromelin. *Indian J. Pharma.* 25:422. (Fights worms.)

Gupta, R. C. et al. 1971. Pharmacognostical study of the leaf of *Calotropis procera* (Ait) R. Br. (Arka). *J. Res. Indian Med.* 6:167–172. (Medicine in the leaves.)

Gupta, R. S. et al. 1990. Calotropin—a novel compound for fertility control. *Anc. Sci. Life 9* (4):224–230.

Hesse, G. et al. 1950. African Arrow Poison. V. Relationship between most important poisons of *Calotropis procera. Justus Liebigs Chem. Annln.* 566:13. (The poisons in the plant.)

Hassal, C. H. and K. Reyle. 1959. Cardenolides. III. Constitution of calatropagenin. *J. Chem. Soc.* 85.

Jain, P. K. et al. 1985. Clinical trial of *arka-mulatwak*—bark of *Calotropis procera*—a preliminary study. *Jour. Res. Ayur. Siddha* 6(1,3 & 4):88–91. (Medicinal properties of the bark.)

Kumar, A. et al. 1990. Pharmacological investigation of flower drug of *Calotropis gigantea* (Asclepiadaceae). Abstract. Manipal: *Proc. 42nd Indian Pharmac. Congr.* p. 87. (Medicinal properties of the flowers.)

Kumar, V. L. et al. 1994. Anti-inflammatory activity of the latex of *Calotropis procera. J. Ethnopharmacol.* 44(2):123–125. (Medicinal value of the milky exudate.)

Murti, P. B. R. and T. R. Seshadri. 1943. Chemical composition of *Calotropis gigantea.* I. Wax and resin components of the latex. *Proc. Indian Acad. Sci.* 18A:146.

———. 1945. Wax and resin components of *Calotropis gigantea.* III. Root bark. *Proc. Indian Acad. Sci.* 21A:147.

———. 1945. Chemical composition of *Calotropis gigantea.* Flowers: a comparison of the composition of the various parts of the plant. *Proc. Indian Acad. Sci.* 22A:304.

Pal, G. and N. K. Sinha. 1980. Isolation, crystallization and properties of calotropins D-I and D-II from *Calotropis gigantea. Archs. Biochem. Biophys.* 202:321. (Enzymes present in the milky exudate.)

Patnaik, G. K. and E. Koechler. 1976. A comparative evaluation of the cardiac effects of asclepin, strophanthin, digoxin and digitoxin. *Indian J. Pharmacol.* 6:11. (Medicines for the heart.)

Prasad, G. 1985. Action of *Calotropis procera* on migraine. *J. Natl. Integ. Med. Assoc.* 27(6):7–10. (A clinical study.)

Qureshi, M. A. et al. 1990. Study on the anti-sperm activity in extracts from different parts of *Calotropis procera. Pak. Jour. Zool.* 23(2):161–165. (Another clinical study.)

Sairam, T. V. 1997. Calotropis, the Unsung Hero. *Dignity Dialogue*, April 15–17.

Shukla, O. P. and C. R. Krishnamurti. 1961. Properties and partial purification of a bacteriolytic enzyme from the latex of *Calotropis procera* (Madar). *J. Sci. Industr. Res.* 20C:109–112.

Singh, B. and R. P. Rastogi. 1972. Structure of asclepin and some observations of NMR spectra of *Calotropis* glycosides. *Phytochemistry* 11:757.

Srivastata, G. N. et al. 1962. Studies on anti-coagulant therapy. Part III. *In vitro* screening of some indian plant latices for fibrinolytic and anticoagulant activity. *Indian J. Med. Sci.* 16:873. (Anti-cancer properties.)

Suresh Kumar, M. and U. K. Chauhan. 1992. A study of anti-microbial activity of *Calotropis procera* leaf extract. *Geobios* 19(2&3):489–490. (Role in fighting germs.)

14

Senna

Cassia senna

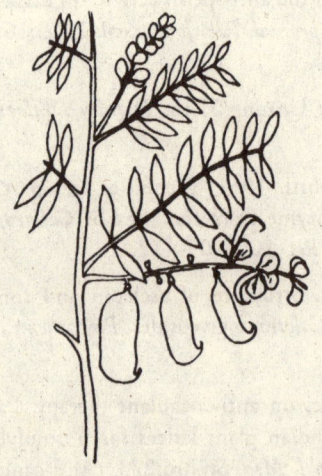

Glory of Medicine

—An Arabic name for
senna

The Gentle Healer

There are two prominent varieties of senna known to Indian
practitioners: Tinnevelly Senna (*Cassia senna*) and Alexandrian
Senna (*Cassia acutifolia*).

American Senna belonging to the same genus grows in the
eastern parts of the United States. The leaves are gathered here
for medicinal use when the plant is in full bloom.

The best variety of senna is obtained from the holy city of
Medina. It is often referred to by hakims as the 'Glory of
Medicine'.

Traditionally, medical practitioners believe that senna

strengthens the heart 'with a feather touch'. The drug is often used as a cathartic in relieving constipation.

The most effective method of ingestion of senna is in the form of tea. Red raisins, violet blossoms, figs, etc. are also added to it. Senna is most often used in purgative decoctions, infusions, powders, pills and enemas.

Profile

Botanical Names	:	*Cassia senna* L. *Cassia angustifolia* Vahl. *Senna alexandrina.*
English Names	:	Senna, Tinnevelly Senna.
Indian Names	:	Hindi : *Senna, Sonamukhi* Malayalam : *Nilavaka* Marathi : *Mulkacha* Tamil : *Nilavirai* Telugu : *Nilaponna* Ayurvedic : *Markandika* Unani : *Sana, Sauna-i-Makki.*
Family	:	Fabaceae.
Sub-family	:	Caesalpinoideae.
Appearance	:	A tall herb with compound leaves, yellowish-green and shiny. Flowers, yellow, arranged in a bunch. Fruit, a flattened legume with compressed seeds.
Distribution	:	The plant is under large scale cultivation in the districts of Tinnevelly (now Tirunelveli), Madurai and Tiruchirapplli in Tamil Nadu.
Other Species	:	*Cassia marilandica* *Cassia acutifolia.*

Medicinal Parts	:	Leaves, pods.
Ayurvedic Preparations	:	*Madhuyashtyadi Churan, Pancha Sakara Churan, Shat Sakara Churan.*
Unani Preparations	:	*Hab Shabyar, Itriffal Mulayyin, Jawarish-ood-Mulayyin, Laooq Sapistan Khiyar Shambari, Sharbat Ahmad Shahi, Sharbat Qabz Kusha, Sufuf Mulliyin.*

In Tradition

AILMENT	PRESCRIPTION
✦ Bad breath, bad taste in the mouth	: Soak 2 tsp senna leaves in 1 glass of boiling water and use the infusion as a mouthwash.
✦ Constipation	: Boil 1 tsp each senna and aniseed in 1 cup of water. While on the boil, add 1 tbsp jaggery. Remove from the fire and drink when warm.
	: Steep 1 tsp senna and 1 tbsp tamarind pulp overnight in 1 cup water and strain in the morning. Add 1 tbsp gulkand (a confection made of rose petals, see chapter on the rose) and eat in the morning.
	: Grind the following into a very fine powder: 1 tsp each fennel, ginger and senna. *Dose:* 1 tsp along with warm water at bedtime.

Note: Individual results may vary.

A Word of Caution

Senna tends to cause griping. To overcome this, some western herbalists recommend its use in combination with figs (which have mild laxative properties) and other carminative and aromatic substances.

In Science

Becker, B. 1959. Active principles of senna. *Planta Med.* 7:390 (Isolated and identified.)

Fairbairn, J. W. 1959. Chemical and pharmacologicval studies on *Cassia acutifolia* and *Rhamnus pushiana. Planta Med.* 7:406; *Chem. Abstr.* 1959.54, 11380.

Fairbairn, J. W. and A. B. Shreshta. 1967. Anthraquinone glycosides. *Phytochemistry* 6:1203.

Fairbairn, J. W. and M. J. R. Moss. 1970. The relative purgative activities of 1, 8-dihydroxyanthracene derivatives. *J. Pharm. Pharmacol.* 22:584. (The purgative activity is attributed to sennosides.)

Lemli, J. and J. Curveele. 1967. Anthraquinone drugs XIV. Isolation of new heterosidic aloe-emodin dianthrone diglucoside from senna leaves. *Pharm. Acta. Helv.* 42:37.

Lust, John. 1974. *The Herb Book.* Bantam Books.

Nattermann, A. and Cie. G.M.B.H. 1969. Sennosides from senna pods. *Britt.* 113528; *Chem. Abstr.* 70, 40626k.

Stoll, A. et al. 1949. The isolation of anthraglycosides from senna drug. *Helv. Chim. Acta.* 32:1892.

Stoll, A. and B. Becker. 1951. Anthraglycosides V. The position of sugar radical in sennosides A and B. *Rec. Trav. Chim.* 69:553; *Chem. Abstr.* 45, 5142f.

Tabin, F. 1914. Constituents of senna leaf. *J. Chem. Soc.* 103:2006.; *Proc. Chem. Soc.* 29:278.

15

Mandukaparni

Centella asiatica

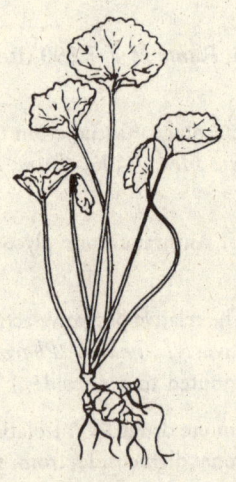

Mandukaparni, a cure for cardiac debility . . .

—Sodhala Nighantu

The Learner's Herb

Mandukaparni in Sanskrit refers to the shape and appearance of leaves of this plant, which resemble the webbed feet of a frog.

The leaves also bear a strong resemblance to the human brain. In conformity with the classical Doctrine of Signature, which postulates that those plants/plant parts that resemble human organs tend to have an impact on them, the drug is believed to affect the mind by reducing mental fatigue and strengthening memory power. Knowing fully well its contribution to the intellect, the Tamil Siddhas have named the herb Saraswati, after the Hindu Goddess of Learning.

The drug has been an ubiquitous ingredient in home remedies for the last three millennia—not only in India but in the entire South East Asian region. The Shaolin priests in China, the Lamas of Tibet, the Japanese, the Indonesians and the Malaysians have all used it as a *kaya-kalpa*, a drug which assures longevity and freedom from the ailments associated with old age.

It is also regarded as a rejuvenator and is said to purify the blood and cure indigestion, nervous weaknesses, vision failures and dysentery. It is recommended in the treatment chronic eczema, secondary and tertiary syphilis with ulceration and leprosy.

The plant contains a chemical, asiaticoside, which is the active agent responsible in curing leprosy. The plant is also considered useful in tuberculosis, elephantiasis, orchitis and other *vata*-aggravations.

Experiments on animals indicate that it promotes the speedy regeneration of hair, nails and skin.

Post-Natal Tonic

The Kotas, a tribal community in Kotagiri in the Nilgiris, use the juice of the leaves as a tonic, particularly for women soon after parturition. It is administered along with palm sugar.

Boon from the Hills

There are two common varieties of mandukaparni: the light green plains-variety and the darker hill-variety. The Siddha physicians prefer the hill variety since it supposedly possesses a higher concentration of active principles.

Profile

Botanical Names	:	*Centella asiatica* (L) Urban. *Hydrocotyle asiatica* Linn.
English Names	:	Indian Pennywort, Gotu Kola.

Indian Names :

Assamese	: *Aghinya*
Bengali	: *Thankhuria*
Gujarati	: *Barmi*
Hindi	: *Brihmi, Brhammanduki,* *Budhbrahmani*
Kannada	: *Urage, Vondelega*
Malayalam	: *Muttil*
Marathi	? *Brahmi*
Punjabi	: *Brahmi-Buti*
Sanskrit	: *Mandukaparni*
Tamil	: *Vallarai*
Telugu	: *Bokkudu, Brahmi,* *Sarasvataku.*

Regional Names :

Naga Hills	: *Aghinya*
Sikkim	: *Gortapri*
Silchar	: *Toonimankoni.*

Family	:	Apiaceae.
Appearance	:	A creeper bearing roots on nodes. Leaves, small, rounded/kidney-shaped, with toothed margins. Flowers, pinkish-red, minute, 3–6 in clusters. Fruits small, 7–9 ridged.
Distribution	:	Throughout India, in moist places, marshy banks of water bodies and irrigated fields.
Medicinal Parts	:	Leaves, roots, seeds, stem, the whole plant.
Drug	:	Fresh and dried leaves and stems.
Preparation	:	Powder, plaster, ointment, waterbath.

106

In Tradition

AILMENT | PRESCRIPTION

🌿 Anaemia : Mix $1/2$ tsp leaf juice with 1 tsp honey and take for 1 month.

🌿 Blockage in blood : Pluck 10 leaves and wash in hot water.
vessels, fatigue, Grind them with 5 black peppercorns.
impairments in Mix into a glass of buttermilk and drink
vision/hearing, on an empty stomach every morning
memory loss, for 3 to 6 months.
symptoms of leprosy,
weakness of heart

🌿 Blurring of vision, : Take $1/4$ tsp *Vallarai Churnam* (powder
muscular fatigue, of the dried leaves) along with honey
nervous weakness, or cow's milk or buttermilk.
sexual debility,
wrinkles in face/skin

🌿 Boils, wounds, : Make a paste of the leaves and apply
swellings on the affected areas.

🌿 Burning sensation : Make a paste of centella and keezhanelli
during urination (*Phyllanthus amarus*) leaves. Take $1/4$
tsp with curd or buttermilk in the
morning.

🌿 Chronic/obstinate : Boil the leaf juice in ghee and apply.
ulcers, eczema,
psoriasis

🌿 Hair loss, : Mix equal quantities of centella leaf
poor memory juice and coconut oil and boil the
mixture well. Cool and bottle. Use as
hair-oil.

❧ Eczema, leprosy, psoriasis

: Boil 3 tsp leaf juice with 3 tsp milk and 1 tsp liquorice powder. Use as an ointment.

❧ Elephantiasis, swellings in neck, etc.

: Fry the required quantity of leaves in castor oil. When lukewarm tie over the affected parts at bedtime.

❧ Fevers, swellings

: Take 4–5 drops of the leaf juice in a cup of cow's milk thrice a day.

❧ Insomnia

: Mix 1/2 tsp powder in 1 cup boiling water. Filter and drink at bedtime.

❧ Leprosy

: Boil a handful of the plant in 1 litre water. Drink the decoction frequently.

❧ Poor memory

: Crush 5 leaves and extract the juice. Mix with 1 tsp honey and take daily.

: Mix dried centella leaves with calamus (16:1) and grind to a very fine powder. *Dose:* 1/4 tsp with honey in the morning and with cow's milk in the evening for 50 days.

❧ Varicose veins

: Mix 1/2 tsp powder in boiling water. Filter and drink.

❧ Venereal diseases, venereal ulcers

: Steam a bunch of leaves and dry them in the shade. When well-dried, powder and store. *Dose:* 1 tsp along with 1 tsp ghee, twice daily.

Note: Individual results may vary.

A Word of Caution

Excess or frequent use may cause body-pain and giddiness.

Instead of using raw leaves as medicine, roasted or boiled leaves are advised.

Mandukaparni: Some Easy Recipes

Centella Powder: A Siddha Medicine

Pluck centella leaves, wash them in hot water and wipe them first with a cloth and then dry them in the shade. For every kilogram of leaves add 100 gm black pepper (for use during winter) or cumin (for use during summer). Grind the mixture into a very fine powder and preserve. *Dosage*: 1/4 tsp every morning on an empty stomach with cow's milk or honey.

Centella Tea

Take 15 fresh centella leaves and boil in 2 cups water till reduced to 1 cup. Add 2 cloves and 2 cardamoms (freshly ground) and 1 tsp honey. Use as a substitute for tea or coffee during the cold season.

Centella Stir Fry

Heat 1 tsp gingelly oil. Add 1/2 tsp mustard seeds and a pinch of asafoetida. When the mustard splutters, add three handfuls of centella leaves and continue frying. Add salt and red chilly powder to taste. When the leaves are cooked, sprinkle with some shredded coconut. Remove from fire after 2 minutes.

This can be eaten as a tasty and nutritious accompaniment to cooked rice or chapattis.

Brahmi or Mandukaparni? A Note

There has been some confusion with regard to the drugs mandukaparni and brahmi mentioned in early Sanskrit texts. Lack of detailed description in the retrieved literature, attribution of the same properties, and use of the same synonyms have all contributed in no small measure. Recently, botanists have more or less agreed to fix the identity of *Bacopa monnieri* (Scrophulariaceae) as *brahmi* and *Centella asiatica* (Apiaceae) as *mandukaparni.*

In Science

Agarwal, S. S. 1981. Some CNS effects of *Hydrocotyle asiatica* Linn. *J. Res. Ayur. Sid.* II. 2:144–149. (Sedative properties of centella.)

Aithal, H. N. and M. Sirsa. 1961. Preliminary pharmacological studies on *Centella asiatica* Linn. *Antiseptic* May, 1961.

Appa Rao, M. V. R. et al. 1967. Six months results of double blind trial to study the effect of *Mandukaparni* and *Punarnava* on normal adults. *J. Vibhuthi Res. Indian Med.* 2:79. (Improves the haemoglobin-content and removes blood-impurities.)

———. 1969. Study of *Mandukaparni* and *Punarnava* for their *rasayana* effect on normal healthy adults. *Nagarjun* 12:33. (Increases blood-protein.)

———. 1973. The effect of *Mandukaparni (Centella asiatica)* on the general mental ability (*medhya*) of mentally retarded children. *J. Res. Indian Med.* 8:9.

Boiteau, P. and A. R. Ratsimamanga. 1956. Asiaticoside extracted from *Centella asiatica*, its therapeutic uses in the healing of experimental or refractory wounds, leprosy, skin tuberculosis and lupus. *Therapie* 11:125–149; *Chem. Abstr.* 51(8):6007h. 1957. (Asiaticoside fights leprosy.)

Central Council for Research in Indian Medicine and Homoeopathy. 1978. *Tribal Pockets of Nilgiris—Recordings of the Field Study on Medicinal Flora and Health Practices.* New Delhi.

Chao, K. H. et al. 1981. Clinical experience of Madecasool (*Centella asiatica*) in the treatment of peptic ulcer. *Korean J. Gastroenterol.* 13(1):49–56. (Effectively treats peptic ulcers.)

Chopra, R. N. et al. 1956. *Glossary of Indian Medicinal Plants.* New Delhi: Council of Scientific and Industrial Research. 58. (Efficacious in the treatment of syphilitic syndromes and tuberculosis.)

Chaudhuri, S. and S. Ghosh. 1977. *Mandukaparni* in the treatment of leprosy. *Bull. Cal. Sch. Trop. Med.* 22(1–4):4–5. (Fights leprosy.)

Dhar, M. L. et al. 1968. Screening of Indian plants for biological activity (Part I). *Indian J. Exp. Bio.* 6(4):232–247. (Antispasmodic properties.)

Jayaweera, M. D. D. 1977. Some Sri Lankan Food Crops and their Medicinal Properties. Colombo: Unesco. *Proceedings of the Third Asian Symposium on Medicinal Plants and Spices.* (A good source of phosphorus, iron, calcium and Vitamin B.)

Handa, S. S. et al. 1986. Natural products and plants as liver-protecting drugs. *Filoterapia* 57(5):307–351.

Hausen, B. M. 1993. *Centella asiatica* (Indian Pennywort)—an effective therapeutic but a weak sensitiser. *Contact Dermatitis* 29(4):175–179.

Malhotra, C. L. et al. 1961. Chemical and pharmacological studies of *Hydrocotyle asiatica* Linn. *Indian J. Pharm.* 23:106. (CNS-depressant activity.)

Patil, J. S. et al. 1998. A study on the immuno stimulation activity of *Centella asiatica* Linn. in rats. *Indian Drugs* 35(11):711–714. (The drug's activity was compared with a potent immuno-stimulant drug, Recombinanant interferon alfa-2b, an adjuant in cancer chemotherapy.)

Rajagopalan, S. S. et al. 1970. Efect of Mandookaparani on growth and tissue composition of albino rats fed on a low protein diet. *Nagarjun* 13:29. (The plant powder administered orally to rats lowered the mortality rate.)

Ramaswamy, A. S. et al. 1970. Pharmacological studies on *Centella asiatica* Linn. (*Brahma Manduki*) (*N. O. Umbelliferae*). *J. Res. Indian Med.* 4:160.

Ramaswamy, A. S. and M. Sirsi. 1960. Antitubercular activity of some chemical constituents from higher plants. *Indian J. Pharm*, 22(2):34–35. (Asiaticoside exhibits antitubercular activity; inhibits the growth of *M. laprae*.)

Rao, A. et al. 1973. The effect of *mandukaparni (Centella asiatica)* on the general mental ability (*medhya*) of mentally retarded children. *J. Res. Indian Med.* 8(4):9–15.

Sharma, A. et al. 1985. Role of *brahmi (Centella asiatica)* in educable mentally-retarded children. *J. Res. Edn. Ind. Med.* 4(1–2):55–57. (Improves memory power.)

Singh, R. H. et al. 1981. Psychotropic effects of *Medhya Rasayana* drug *Mandukaparni (Hydrocotyle asiatica)*. Part III. *J. Res. Ayur. Siddha* 2(1):110. (Cure for anxiety-neurosis.)

Sukh Dev. 1983. Natural products in medicine—present status and future prospects. *Curr. Sci.* 52(20):947–956.

Usman Ali, S. et al. 1981. Contribution to the exact botanical identity of *brahmi* and *mandukaparni*. *Bull. Med. Ethnobot. Res.* 2(1):23–36.

16

Bone-Setter

Cissus quadrangularis

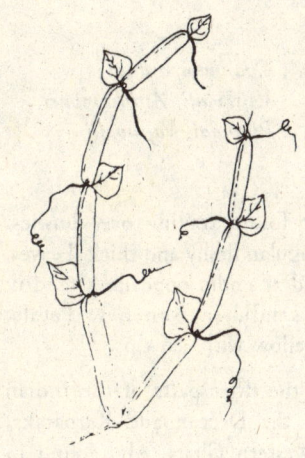

*Ghritakumari, cooling, bitter
. . . a fighter of pitta*

—Raja Nighantu

Herbal Cement

The ubiquitous painted signboards advertising the bone healer's arts in Indian cities are sadly enough, the only reminders of a long healing tradition based on common herbs. Foremost among these is an oddly-shaped climber, whose name in Sanskrit, *Asthisamhari* and its English rendering, the Bone-Setter convey its folk use in the treatment of broken bones.

The tribal belts of Bihar, Gujarat, Madhya Pradesh, Maharashtra and Rajasthan have all borne witness to the contribution of this plant in setting right all types of skeletal fractures, bone and muscle injuries, sprains, muscular pains and contusions in limbs from prehistoric times.

Experiments conducted in Indian laboratories have upheld the traditional use of this plant as an analgesic.

Profile

Botanical Names	:	*Cissus quadrangularis* L. *Vitis quadrangularis* (L) Wallich ex Wight
Indian Names	:	Malayalam : *Channamparanta* Sanskrit : *Vajravalli, Asthisamhari* Tamil : *Pirandai, Vajravalli.*
Family	:	Vitaceae.
Appearance	:	A climber found trailing over bushes. Stem, 4-angular, fleshy and thick. Leaves, oval, found at nodes opposite a tendril. Flowers, small, in bunches. Petals, greenish yellow with red tips.
Distribution	:	Found in the drier parts of the Indian peninsula: the Deccan and Karnataka, and the Western Ghats. Also found in the drier regions of Africa and Arabia.
Medicinal Parts	:	The whole plant.
Ayurvedic Preparations	:	*Pathya Punarnavadi Kashayam, Valiya Chichadi Leham.*

In Tradition

AILMENTS	PRESCRIPTION
❧ Amenorrhoea, painful menstruation	: Take a pinch or two of the ash (See below) along with 1 tsp ghee. Three times a day for 3–4 days.

114

✤ Diarrhoea	: Add a pinch of the ash to a little hot water and drink.
✤ Fatigue, nervous weakness, sexual debility, stomach ailments	: Take a pinch of the ash along with a pinch of nutmeg. Mix the powders with 1 tsp ghee and eat 3 times a day for a week.
✤ Injuries, muscular pain, sprains	: Grind the whole plant into a fine paste with equal quantities of fresh turmeric rhizomes. Apply generously on the affected parts. Bandage and leave undisturbed for a few days.
✤ Obesity	: Take 2 to 3 pinches of the ash along with buttermilk or coconut water.
✤ Piles, stomach ailments, ulcer	: Take 2 to 3 pinches of the ash with 1 tsp ghee continuously for 2 months.
✤ Stomach ache	: Take a handful each of the whole bone-setter plant and drumstick flowers along with 1 tbsp copra (dried coconut). Grind with a little water and extract the juice. Drink.
✤ Swelling due to injuries	: Crush the plant and extract 1 cup juice. Add 1 tsp each salt and tamarind and boil the mixture. While bearably hot, apply on the affected areas.

Note: Individual results may vary.

Ash of Bone-Setter

In the Siddha system, certain plant substances often undergo a

115

process by which they are burnt into ash before being employed as medicine. The bone-setter is an ideal example of this method. The village vaidyar in South India crushes the plant thoroughly and mixes it with common salt (3:1 ratio) before placing it between two identical, concave clay bowls. Having ensured the proper sealing of the crevice between the juxtaposed bowls with the help of an ingenious sealing compound—either a paste of wheat flour or a cloth dipped in a red earth and water mixture and dried, and then tied around the crevice—the contraption is fired. Normally it is dried cow dung cakes alone which are used in the kiln. When the firing is complete, the two halves of the bowl are separated and the grey-coloured ash-remnants of the bone-setter is obtained. This is stored in a bottle for use as and when required.

A Word of Caution

The juice of the plant can irritate the skin; it may cause itching. The bone-setter's ash, in excess can be toxic. Self-medication or frequent use could prove harmful.

In Science

Chopra, S. S. et al. 1975. Studies of *Cissus quadrangularis* in experimental fracture repair. Effect on chemical parameters in blood. *Indian J. Med. Res.* 63(5):824–828. (Cardiotonic characteristics of the plant.)

———. 1976. Studies of *Cissus quadrangularis* in experimental fracture repair. A histopathological study. *Indian J. Med. Res.* 64(9):1365–1368.

Dhar, M. L. et al. 1968. Screening of Indian plants for biological activity. Part I. *Indian J. Exptl. Biol.* 6:232. (Anti-amoebic properties of the plant reported.)

Das, P. K. and A. K. Sanyal. 1964. Studies on *Cissus quadrangularis*

Linn. Part I. Acetylcholine like action of the total extract. *Indian J. Med. Res.* 52:63. (Ethanolic extract produced acetylcholine like activity on isolated smooth muscle preparations and ileum of rabbits etc.)

Dhawan, B. N. et al. 1980. Screening of Indian plants for biological activity. Part IX. *Indian J. Exptl. Biol.* 18(6):594–606. (The plant could regularize irregular menstruation problems.)

Ekanayake, D. T. 1980. Plants used in the treatment of skeletal fractures in indigenous system of medicine in Sri Lanka. *Sri Lanka For.* 14(3&4): 45–152.

Jain, S. K. and C. R. Tarafdar. 1970. *Medicinal Plantlore of Santhals.* *Econ. Bot.* 24(3): 241–278.

Maheswari, Y. K. et al. 1986. Ethno-medicine of Bhil tribe of Jhabua Dist. M. P. *Ancient Sci. Life.* 5(4):255–261.

Misra, S. B. and S. N. Dixit. 1979. Antifungal activity of leaf extracts of some higher plants. *Acta Bot. Indica* 7(2): 147–150. (Fungicidal activity of leaf extract reported.)

Prasad, G. C. and K. N. Udupa. 1963. Effect of *Cissus quadrangularis* on the healing of cortisone treated fractures. *Indian J. Med. Res* 51(4): 667–676. (The mechanism of healing of fractures: the extract neutralized the anti-anabolic effect of cortisone treated fractures and enhanced healing. The stimulatory effect of the extract was much greater than the well-known anabolic hormone, durabolin.)

————. 1970. Role of *Cissus quadrangularis* on fracture healing. Varanasi: Banaras Hindu University. *Advances in Research in Indian Medicine.* 163.

————. 1970 Effect of phytogenic steroid of *Cissus quadrangularis* (Hadjora) on endocrine glands after fracture. *J. Res. Indian Med.* 4:132. (How the plant cures fractures.)

————. 1972. Pathways and site of action of phytogenic steroid from *Cissus quadrangularis.* *J. Res. Indian Med.* 7:29.

Sen, S. P. 1966. Studies on active constituents of *Cissus quadrangularis.* *Curr. Sci.* 35(12):317.

Subbu, V. S. V. 1968. Pharmacological evaluation of a glucoside obtained from the plant *Vitis quadrangularis. Indian J. Physiol. Pharmacol.* 12:5. (Intravenous administration of a water soluble crystalline glucoside isolated from the stem exhibited hypotensive response in dogs.)

————. 1970. Pharmacological and toxicological evaluation of an active principle obtained from the plant *Vitis quadrangularis. Indian J. Pharmac.* 2:91.

————. 1971. Mechanism of action of Vitis glucoside on myocardial tissue. *Indian J. Med. Sc.* 25:400.

Udupa, K. N. and G. C. Prasad. 1964. Biochemical and Ca 45 studies on the effect of *Cissus quadrangularis* in fracture healing. *Indian J. Med. Res.* 52:480. (The studies indicated early completion of calcification and 90% gain in normal strength in 1 month.)

————. 1965. The effect of phytogenic, anabolic steroid in the acceleration of fracture repair. *Life Sci.* 4:317. (An anabolic steroid isolated from the plant proved potent in fracture healing as evidenced by its influence at an accelerated rate on the early regression of all connective tissue cells involved in the healing and mineralization of the callus.)

17

Kovai

Coccinia indica

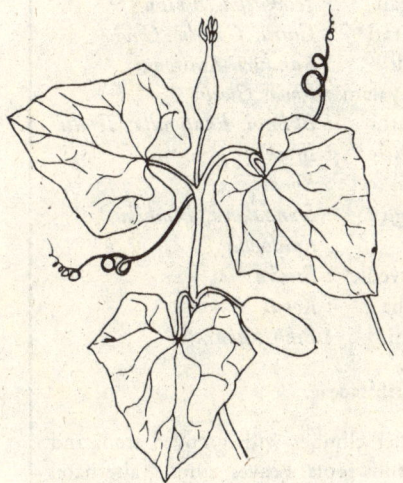

The fruit of bimbi is useful in the treatment of breathing problems . . .

—Dhanavantari Nighantu

Plant of Many Parts

Kovai fruits are widely used as a vegetable in many parts of the country, and native physicians and housewives have been using them as a household remedy for various ailments. It is frequently used as a cure for diabetes. The presence of certain enzymes in the juice is believed to rapidly hydrolyse starch. It is also employed to cure a host of other diseases: convulsions, cough, dyspepsia, emaciation, fevers accompanied by a burning sensation, infective hepatitis, menorrhagia, scrofula, syphilis, ulcers, etc.

In several Indian village schools, the leaves of kovai are used as a duster to clean slates and blackboards.

Profile

Botanical Names	:	*Coccinia grandis* (L) Voigt
		Coccinia cordifolia (L) Cogn.
		Coccinia indica Wt. & Arn.
		Cephalandra indica Naud. C.
English Names	:	Covel, Kovai, Scarlet Gourd.

Indian Names :

Bengali	:	*Telakucha, Bimbu*
Gujarati	:	*Gluru, Galedu, Ghobe*
Hindi	:	*Kanduri, Kudroom*
Malayalam	:	*Kova, Gwel*
Marathi	:	*Bhimbi, Rantondla, Tendli*
Sanskrit	:	*Bimbi*
Tamil	:	*Kovai*
Telugu	:	*Dondakaya, Bimbika, Kaidonda*
Ayurvedic	:	*Bimba*
Siddha	:	*Kovai*
Unani	:	*Bikh Kabar.*

Family	:	Cucurbitaceae.
Appearance	:	Slender climber with grooved stem and tuberous roots. Leaves, simple, alternate, 3 to 5 lobed, shiny. Flowers, solitary, white, unisexual. Fruit oval and ellipsoid, slightly beaked, green with white stripes and bright red when ripe. Seeds compressed, glandular.
Distribution	:	Cultivated in Assam, Bihar, Orissa, Bengal, Maharashtra, Andhra Pradesh and Tamil Nadu.
Medicinal Parts	:	Stem, fruit, leaf, root, bark.
Ayurvedic Preparations	:	*Amritaprasa Ghritam, Vastyamayantaka Ghritam, Vidaryadi Ghritam* and *Kashayam.*

In Tradition

AILMENTS	PRESCRIPTION

❧ Animal-bites, skin eruptions, sores : Apply a fresh paste of leaves on the affected areas.

❧ Body-heat : Extract the juice from the leaves. Take 5 tsp along with 1 glass water thrice daily for 3 days.

❧ Body-heat, burning eyes, psoriasis, skin infections : Boil 1 cup leaves in 1 cup water till the volume is reduced by half. Drink.

: Dry some leaves and grind them into a fine powder. Store in a glass bottle in a cool place. Mix 1 tsp powder in hot water and drink thrice a day.

❧ Body-heat, diabetes, dryness of the skin : Eat two fruits (raw) every day.

❧ Body-heat, psoriasis, skin infections : Boil 1 cup leaf juice with an equal quantity of gingelly oil till the mixture is reduced to half the original quantity. Cool and bottle. Apply this on the affected areas or massage all over the body.

❧ Diabetes : Take 1 tsp juice of the roots with 1 cup water. (*Note:* 1. This treatment can be a supplement to other treatments for diabetes such as diet-based therapy, etc. 2. In a laboratoy experiment conducted by the Central Research

Institute for Siddha, Trivandrum, it was recorded that the root did not show any hypoglycaemic activity, although the fruits were found to be usually more potent.)

❧ Diarrhoea : Extract the juice from the leaves. Mix 2 tsp juice with $1/2$ cup curd and take twice or thrice daily.

❧ Inflammation : Fry a handful of leaves in neem oil. When bearably hot, apply on the swelling and bandage.

❧ Obesity : Boil 2 tsp stem in 1 cup water till the volume is reduced by half. Drink.

❧ Painful eyes : Extract the juice from the leaves. Instil 2 drops in the eyes thrice daily for 3 days. (*Caution:* Take precautions to prevent infection while handling.)

❧ Scabies : Extract $1/2$ cup juice from leaves. Add 1 tsp butter and mix thoroughly. Apply on the affected parts frequently.

❧ Sores on the tongue : Chew the tender fruits for at least 10 minutes.

❧ Urine blockage : Boil 2 tsp roots in 1 cup water till the water is reduced by half. Drink.

Note: Individual results may vary.

In Science

Bhakuni, D. S. et al. 1962. Chemical examination of the fruits of *Coccinia indica*. *J. Sci. Industr. Res.* 21B:237–238.

Bisht, B. S. and S. L. Nayar. 1958. Pharmacognosy of root and leaf of *Coccinia indica* Wight & Arn. *Journal Sci. Ind. Res.* 17C:45–51.

Brahmachari, H. D. and K. T. Augusti. 1965. Orally effective hypoglycaemic principles from *Coccinia indica*. *J. Pharm. & Pharma.* 15(6):417.

Chatterjee, M. 1991. Study of hypoglycaemic activity of indigenous medicinal plants in experimental diabetic animal models. University of Calcutta: doctoral thesis.

Chopra, R. N. et al. 1956. *Glossary of Indian Medicinal Plants.* New Delhi: CSIR. p. 72. (The drug is prescribed for skin eruptions; internally for gonorrhoea.)

Chowdhury, R. R. and M. Mishra. 1987. *Coccinia indica* in type II diabetes mellitus. *Indian Med. Jour.* 81(2):31–32.

Chowdhury, R. R. and S. B. Vohora. 1970. Plants with possible hypoglycaemic activity. *Advances in Res. in Indian Med.* Varanasi: Banaras Hindu University. 57.

Das, A. 1976–77. Bitters and Diabetes. *Indian Drugs* 14:168. (Compared to exogenous insulin and synthetic drugs, this drug is of limited value; it is likely that the drug induces production of gastric juice and the flow of intestinal hormones, which in turn activate release of insulin.)

De, N. N. and B. Mukherjee. 1953. Effect of *Coccinia indica* Wight & Arn. on alloxan diabetes in rabbits (A preliminary note). *Indian J. Med Sci.* 7:665–672. (Water-soluble alkaloid obtained from alcoholic extract of the root exhibited anti-diabetic property.)

Gupta, S. S. 1963. Experimental studies on pituitary diabetes. Part II. Effect of indigenous anti-diabetic drugs against the acute hyperglycaemic response of anterior pituitary extract in glucose-fed albino rats. *Indian J. Med. Res.* 51:716. (The plant extract produced appreciable inhibition.)

Gupta, S. S. and M. C. Variyar. 1964. Experimental studies on pituitary diabetes. Part IV. Effect of *Gymnaema sylvestre* and *Coccinia indica* against the acute hyperglycaemic response of somatotropin and corticotropin hormones. *Indian J. Med. Res.* 52:2000. (Alcoholic extract of the plant exhibited significant hypoglycaemic effect.)

Khan Azad, A. K. et al. 1980. Treatment of Diabetes mellitus with *Coccinia indica. Brit. Med. Jour.* 280(6220):1044.

Kuppurajan, K. et al. 1986. Hypoglycaemic effect of *Coccinia indica* in Diabetes mellitus. *Nagarjun* 29(5):1–4.

Mukherjee, B. 1962. Drug Research. *Eastern Pharmacist* 5:35. (Clinical trials reveal that the drug is of limited value in controlling diabetes as compared to exogenous insulin or synthetic drugs.)

Mukherjee, K. et al. 1972. Preliminary observation on pharmacological properties of a water-soluble alkaloid of *Coccinia indica* Linn. Part I. *Indian J. Pharmac.* 4:114. (Both single dose as well as chronic oral administration of extracts of the whole plant and leaf showed significant hypoglycaemic action.)

Patra, B. B. et al. 1975. Pharmacological studies with *Coccinia indica. Annual Conference Assoc. Physiol. and Pharmacol. of India.*

Pillai, N. R. et al. 1980. Hypoglycaemic activity of *Coccinia indica* W & A. *Bull. Med. Ethnobot. Res.* 1(2):234–242.

Rajasekharan, S. et al. 1984. Clinical evaluation of Siddha drugs in the treatment of Manjal Kamalai (infective hepatitis) Part I. Kovai (*Coccinia grandis* W & A). *J. Res. Ayur. Siddha* 5(1–4):18–24.

Ramachandran, K. and B. Subramanian. 1983. Scarlet gourd, *Coccinia grandis*, little known tropical drug plant. *Econ. Bot.* 37:380. (The juice extracted from stems, leaves and roots alone or as a tablet made from homogenized and freeze-dried leaves is used to treat glycosuria.)

Satyavati et al. 1976. *Medicinal Plants of India.* New Delhi. Vols. I & II. p. 262. (Pharmacognosy of the plant, *Coccinia indica.*)

Sikdar, S. et al. 1972. Pharmacological studies with a water-soluble alkaloid of *Coccinia indica.* Jaipur: *Fifth Annual Conference Indian Pharmacol. Soc.*

_____ 1975. Studies on the hypoglycaemic property of a water-soluble alkaloid of *Coccinia indica* Linn. *Calcutta Medical Club Journal.*

18

Guggul

Commiphora mukul

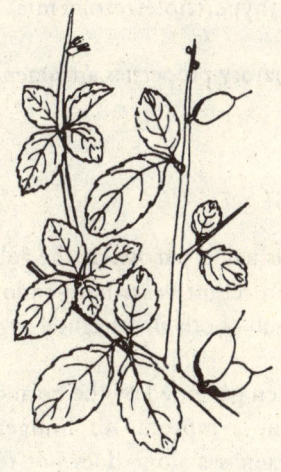

Guggulu protects against curses.

—Atharva Veda

Commoner of Vedic Times

The Atharva Veda, the seminal source of Ayurveda, has described guggul vividly. The plant which is worshipped in Indian villages presents an unassuming profile: a shrub growing in arid, rocky wastelands, with hungry outstretched branches and sparing leaves.

Strong-Smelling Gum

Guggul is the source of Indian Bdellium, a gum exuded by the plant during the harsh summer months. It is dull green or brown in colour with a balsamic odour and a bitter aromatic taste. The gum is popularly used as an incense to fumigate rooms. Besides its aromatic properties, such fumigation has an antiseptic effect. The gum, used widely in native medicine, is astringent and antiseptic.

Recent scientific tests have upheld the traditional use of the gum: its role in combating arthritis, as well as its role in the prevention and rolling back of hypercholesterolaemia and ischaemic heart-diseases.

Its well recognized anti-inflammatory properties are amenable to easy bottling and storage.

The Goblin and His Uses

The gum fights obesity too, hence its name, *palankusa,* the goblin. Scientific experiments conducted in recent years have endorsed the hypolipidaemic action of guggul—both in its crude as well as extractive forms.

Fat metabolism, we know, is often governed by the hormones in obese people. Perpetuating the symptoms of hunger or torturing one's limbs with tiring exercises alone does not result in slimmer bodies. In this context, it is interesting that guggul can offer a way out: it can engage effectively with hormone-induced obesity as well. Clinical experiments conducted on guggul's impact on obese people have raised the hopes of many a drooping spirit: sustained weight-reduction at an average of 2% per month has been recorded.

Freshly gathered guggul is considered to be an aphrodisiac and tonic. According to Sushruta, it is the guggul that is stored which can help in reducing obesity and corpulency.

Profile

Botanical Names	:	*Commiphora wightii* (Arn) Bhand.
		Commiphora mukul (Hook ex Stocks)
		Balsamodendron roxburghii Stocks

Indian Names	:	Hindi, Bengali &
		Gujarati : *Guggul, Mukul*
		Marathi &
		Kannada : *Guggule*
		Sanskrit : *Divya, Durga, Kumbha,*
		Siva, Ambahava, Usha
		Tamil : *Gukkulu, Maishakshi*
		Telugu : *Gugul, Mahisaksh,*
		Maisakshi
		Ayurvedic : *Guggulu*
		Unani : *Guggal.*

Family : Burseraceae.

Appearance : A slow-growing shrub with knotty, spiny branches. Leaflets 1–3, toothed. Flowers brownish red. Fruits, red. The cut surface of the plant secretes a gum, which is a lustrous, pale brown, semi-solid mass.

Distribution : Grows wild in the rocky, arid areas of Kathiawar, Karnataka and Rajasthan.

Medicinal Parts : Oleoresin (gum).

Ayurvedic Preparations : *Yogaraja Guggulu, Kaisore, Navka Guggulu, Vasa Guggulu, Amritadya Guggulu, Triphala Guggulu, Simhanada Guggulu,* etc.

Unani Preparations : *Hab Mugil, Zimad Bawasir, Marham Ushaq.*

Other Species : *Commiphora myrrha* yields myrrh, which is used in toothpaste and perfumes. The oil is antiseptic and anti-inflammatory.

In Tradition

AILMENT	PRESCRIPTION
❧ Anaemia, liver diseases, obesity, skin diseases	: Take 1/4 tsp guggul powder along with honey and lime juice on an empty stomach in the morning.
❧ Bronchitis, hay fever, laryngitis, nasal catarrh	: Burn the gum and inhale the fumes.
❧ Caries of the teeth, pyorrhoea, ulcerated throat, weak and spongy gums	: Mix 1/2 tsp guggul powder in 1 glass warm water. Use as a mouthwash and gargle.
❧ Dyspepsia, indigestion, loss of appetite	: Take 1/4 tsp guggul powder with 1/2 cup lukewarm water half an hour before a meal.
❧ Obesity	: Take 1/4 tsp guggul powder along with hot water 3 or 4 times a day.
❧ Uclers, wounds	: Mix the gum in a little coconut oil and apply on the wounds.

Note: Individual results may vary.

In Science

Ahuja, M. M. S. et al. 1977. Effect of fraction 'A' of *Commiphora mukul* on Mangolian gerbils (*Meriones unguiculatus*). *Indian J. Exptl. Biol.* 15(2):143–145. (Lowers cholesterol.)

Amma, M. K. P. et al. 1978. Effect of oleoresin of Gum Guggulu (*Commiphora mukul*) on the reproductive organs of female rats. *Indian J. Exptl. Biol.* 16(9):1021–1023. (Anti-fertility properties noted.)

Arora R. B. et al. 1971. Chemical and pharmacological approach of a pure steroid from an indigenous herb, *Commiphora* (Gum Guggulu) with special reference to its hypolipidemic activity. New Delhi: *Paper presented in the Seminar on Disorders of Lipid Metabloism and the Role of Guggulu (C. mukul) as a Therapeutic Agent.* Oct. 1971. (Fights obesity.)

————. 1971. Isolation of crystalline steroidal compound from *C. mukul* and its anti-inflammatory action. *Indian J. Exp. Biol.* 9:403. (Anti-inflammatory efficacy recorded.)

————. 1973. Effect of some fractions of *C. mukul* on various serum lipid levels in hypercholestrolemic chicks and their effectiveness in myocardial infarction in rats. *Indian J. Exp. Biol.* Vol II. (Solves cholesterol problems and myocardial infarction.)

Arora, R. B. et al. 1977. Isolation of a crystalline steroid compound from *Commiphora mukul* and its anti-inflammatory activity. *Indian J. Exptl. Biol.* 9(3):403–404.

————. 1982. Beneficial effect of fraction 'A' of Gum Guggulu in arthritic syndrome of liver function in clinical and experimental arthritis. *Rheumatism* 18(1):9–16. (Effective against arthritis.)

Bagi, M. K. et al. 1985. Preliminary pharmacological studies of essential oil from *Commiphora mukul. Filoterapia* 56:245. (Depressant action on the heart.)

Bhatt, B. 1987. Effect of katibasti in sciatica. *Rheumatism* 22:61. (Effective in sciatica.)

Bhatti, A. J. 1950. Essential oil from the resin of *C. Mukul. J. Indian Chem. Soc.* 27:436.

Bordia, A. and S. K. Chutani. 1979. Effect of gum guggulu on fibrinolysis and platelette adhesiveness in coronary heart-disease. *Indian J. Med. Res.* 70:992–996. (Cholesterol-lowering properties.)

Bose, S. and K. C. Gupta. 1962. Structure of *Commiphora mukul* gum: Part I. Nature of sugars present and structure of aldobiouronic acid. *Indian J. Chem.* 2:57.

Chopra, R. N. et al. 1956. *Glossary of Indian Medicinal Plants.* New Delhi: Council of Scientific and Industrial Research. (In the treatment of snakebite and scorpion sting.)

Dennis, T. J. et al. 1980. Pharmacognostic study of the gum oleo-resin of *Commiphora wightii. Bull. Med. Ethnobot. Res.* 1:72.

Dutt, A. T. et al. 1942. Chemical investigation of gum-resin from *Balsamodendron mukul. Indian J. Med. Res.* 30:331.

Jha, S. D. and V. N. Pandey. 1985. Clinical study on 'Kitebh' (Psoriasis). *J. Res. Ayur. Siddha* 6(2)195–212. (Effective against psoriasis.)

Kakrani, H. K. 1981. Flavanoids from the flowers of *Commiphora mukul. Filoterapia* 52:221.

————. 1981. *In vitro* antimicrobial activity of essential oil of *Commiphora mukul* and *Commiphora roxburghii. Bull. Med. Ethnobot. Res.* 2:100. (Antibacterial and antifungal activities.)

Kakrani, H. K. and G. A. Kalyani. 1984. Anthelmintic activity of essential oil of *Commiphora mukul. Filoterapia* 55:232. (Kills tapeworms and hookworms more efficiently than piperazine phosphate and hexyl resorcinol respectively.)

Kappurajan, K. et al. 1973. Effect of guggulu (*Commiphora mukul*) in serum lipids in obese subjects. *J. Res. Indian Med.* 8(4):1–8. (Significant decrease in serum cholesterol levels.)

Khanna, D. S. et al. 1969. Biochemical approach to anti-arteriosclerotic action of *Commiphora mukul,* an indigenous drug in Indian domestic pigs *(Sus crofa). Indian J. Med. Res.* 57(5):900–906.

Kotiyal, J. P. et al. 1979. Double blind cross over trial of *Commiphora mukul* (Fraction 'A') in hypercholesterolaemia and obesity. *J. Res. Indian Med. Yoga and Homoeo.* 14(2):11–16. (Brings down cholesterol levels.)

Majumdar, A. 1979. Selection of the drugs for trial in rheumatoid arthritis. *Rheumatism* 14(2):53–76. (Usefulness in liver disorders and hemiplagia.)

Mahta, V. L. et al. 1968. The effect of various fractions of gum guggulu on experimentally produced hypercholesterolemia in chicks. *Indian J. Physiol. Pharmacol.* 12:91–95. (Proof of its cholesterol-lowering action.)

Malhotra, S. C. et al. 1977. Long term clinical studies on the hypolipidaemic effect of *Commiphora mukul* and Clofibrate. *Indian J. Med. Res.* 65(3):390–395.

Mickelson, O. 1955. Experimental obesity Part I. Production of obesity in rats by feeding high fat diets. *J. Nutrition* 57:541.

Nityanand, S. et al. 1973. Cholestrol activity of various fractions of *Commiphora mukul* (guggul). *Indian J. Pharmacol.* 5:259.

————. 1971. Hypocholesterolemic effect of *C. Mukul* resin. *Indian J. Exp. Biol.* 9:376. (Controls cholesterol.)

————. 1973. Cholesterol-lowering activity of various fractions of *Commiphora mukul* (Guggul). *Indian J. Pharmacol.* 5:259.

————. 1975. Hypolipidaemic effect of ethylacetate fraction of *Commiphora mukul* (Guggul) in rats. *Indian J. Pharmacol.* 13:755.

Pandit, M. M. and C. P. Shukla. 1981. Study of Siddha guggulu on rheumatoid arthritis. *Rheumatism* 16(2):54–57. (Fights arthritis.)

Patil, V. D. et al. 1972. Chemistry of Ayurvedic Drugs. I. Guggulu. (resin from *Commiphora mukul*) steroidal constituents. *Tetrahedron* 28:2341.

Prem Kishore et al. 1990. Clinical studies on the treatment of Amavata (rheumatoid arthritis) with Sunthi Guggulu. *J. Res. Ayur. Siddha* 3(3&4):133–146.

Purushothaman, K. K. and S. Chandrasekharan. 1976. Guggulsterols from *Commiphora mukul. Indian J. Chem.* 14b:802.

Santhakumari, G. et al. 1964. Further studies on the anti-arthritic and anti-inflammatory activities of gum guggul. *Indian J. Physiol. Pharmacol.* 8:36. (Lowering of serum and tissue lipids.)

Satyavati, G. V. and S. N. Tripathi. 1966. Effect of an indigenous drug (Guggulu) on disorders of lipid metabolism with special reference to arteriosclerosis and obesity. Borochure. Varanasi: P.G.I.I.M. Banares Hindu University. p. 77. (Role in arteriosclerosis and obesity documented.)

———— 1969. *C. Mukul* Engl. and *Tinospora cordifolia* Willd.—A study of anti-inflammatory activity. *Rheumatism* 4:141.

————. 1969. Experimental studies on the hypocholesterolemic effect of *Commiphora mukul* (guggul). *Indian J. Med. Res.* 57(10):1950–1962.

Sharma, S. D. et al. 1986. New Ayurvedic compound for management of ischaemic heart-diseases. *Ancient Sci. Life* 5(3):161–167. (As a cure for cardiac ischaemia.)

Singh, A. K. et al. 1985. Hormonal response of thyroid gland to *Commiphora mukul* and LATS in tissue culture. *Bull. Medico-Ethno-Bot. Res.* 6(4):155–164. (Stimulates the thyroid.)

Sukh Dev. 1983. Chemistry of resinous exudates of some Indian trees. *Proc. Indian Natn. Sci. Acad.* 49A:359.

Swarn. et al. 1972. Cholesterol lowering activity of the various fractions of guggulu. *Indian J. Exp. Biol.* II:5:395–397.

Tripathi, S. N. et al. 1968. Experimental and clinical studies on the effect of Guggulu (*C. Mukul*) in hyperlipimia and thrombosis. *J. Res. Indian Med.* 3:2.

———— 1975. Effect of keto-steroid of *Commiphora mukul* E. on hypercholesterolemia and hyperlipidaemia induced by neomercazole and cholesterol mixture in chicks. *Indian J. Exp. Biol.* 13(1):15–18.

Tripathi, V. 1999. Preventive and curative aspects of a herbal formulation (Atherocid) in the management of Ischaemic Heart Disease (IHD). New Delhi: *Second International Symposium on Cardiovascular Surgery and Cardiology.* (The drug is a combination of 7 herbs: arjuna, guggul, jalneem, kut, prishnaparni, pushkarmool and shankhpushpi.)

Tripathi, Y. B. et al. 1984. Thyroid stimulating action of z-guggulsterone obtained from *Commiphora mukul. Planta Med.* 50:78. (Strong thyroid stimulating action when administered to albino rats.)

Vyas, S. N. and C. P. Shukla. 1987. A clinical study on the effect of Shuddha Guggulu in rheumatoid arthritis. *Rheumatism* 23:15. (As an analgesic and in rheumatoid arthritis.)

19

Durva

Cynodon dactylon

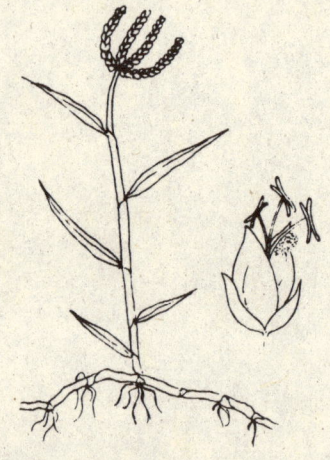

Durva, one of the ten complexion-promoters .

—Charaka

Green Blood

In recent times, in certain parts of Tamil Nadu, the health-conscious population has begun to make a beeline for their latest in a cuppa—*arugampull* juice. Full of chlorophyll, durva juice which contains many vital, nourishing factors has come to be revered as 'green blood'.

The traditional Siddha system sings its praise as 'the remover of toxins'. Ayurveda calls it *sahasravirya* denoting its versatility and vitality.

The drug is a reputed remedy in epistaxis (*nasagada-rakta-pittam*), hematuria and scabies. It is cooling, astringent, demulcent, diuretic, ophthalmic, haemostatic and suppurative.

Profile

Botanical Names	:	*Cynodon dactylon* (L.) Pers.
		Panicum dactylon Linn.
English Names	:	Bahamas Grass, Bermuda Grass, Doob Grass.
Indian Names	:	Hindi : *Doob*
		Kannada : *Garikehulla*
		Malayalam : *Karuka, Karukappullu*
		Sanskrit : *Ananta, Devika, Durva*
		Tamil : *Arugampul, Muthandam, Thurvai*
		Telugu : *Gericha Gaddi.*
Family	:	Gramineae (Poaceae).
Appearance	:	A perennial grass, used as fodder. Stem, slender, creeping, rooting at all nodes; branches, erect; leaves, narrowly linear; fruit, oblong, laterally compressed grain.
Distribution	:	A very common weed throughout India and in the tropical and warm temperate regions throughout the world. It is also one of the commonest grasses used on tennis lawns.
Medicinal Parts	:	Roots, the whole plant.

In Tradition

AILMENT	PRESCRIPTION

❧ Bleeding piles

: Crush 2 tbsp cleaned, fresh grass. Add 1 teacup cow's milk and boil. Filter and drink.

: Grind equal quantities of grass with roots into a fine paste. Boil 1 tbsp in 1 cup cow's milk and drink.

❧ Blood-discharges from mouth, nose, ear, eye, urinary tract, anus, etc., excess menstruation

: Boil $1/2$ cup clean grass with an equal quantity of the tender leaves of pomegranate in 2 cups of water till reduced to 1 cup. Strain and cool. *Dose:* $1/2$ cup. Repeat after 2 hours.

❧ Blood in urine, burning sensation during urination, dryness of skin

: Grind 2 tbsp cleaned grass along with 1 tbsp keezhanelli into a fine paste. Add 1 cup diluted buttermilk. Drink every morning.

❧ Body-heat, burning sensation in eyes, burning sensation during urination, diarrhoea

: Boil 3 tbsp pulp of ash-gourd along with 3 tbsp cleaned grass in 2 cups of water till the volume is reduced to 1 cup. *Dose:* $1/2$ cup thrice a day.

❧ Breathing problems, congestion in lungs, phlegm

: Crush 2 tbsp cleaned grass along with 10 black peppercorns and boil in 2 cups of water till the volume is reduced to 1 cup. *Dose:* $1/2$ cup 3–4 times a day.

❧ Cholesterol in blood, lipid accumulation in blood vessels, obesity

: Make a paste of 2 tbsp grass, 6 black peppercorns and 2 pinches of cumin. Take twice a day along with buttermilk or coconut water.

✤ Cuts, wounds	: Grind the grass and garlic (4:1 ratio) into a fine paste and apply. Bandage firmly.
✤ Eye-ailments; to strengthen eyesight	: Extract the pure sap of the cleaned grass and use as eye drops. (*Caution:* Take all necessary precautions to prevent infection.)
✤ Eye-ailments, headache	: Soak a handful of leaves in 1 teacup water. Strain. Add 1 tbsp milk. Drink with or without sugar.
✤ Heart-diseases	: Boil 1 tbsp crushed tender grass in 1 cup water and take twice daily for 7 days.
✤ Sunstroke, prevention of stress and strain	: Dry the grass and grind into a fine powder. Bottle. *Dose:* Boil 1/2 tsp powder in water. Add milk and a little sugar and take as a substitute for tea or coffee, twice daily.
✤ Heaviness in the head	: Grind together cynodon, white garlic, rice and leaves of cucumber. Apply over the forehead.
	: Grind together cynodon, rice and long chillies. Boil the paste. Apply over the forehead.
✤ Infection in between the toes, prickly heat, psoriasis, skin-infections	: Grind cleaned grass without the roots and turmeric (4:1) into a fine paste and apply on the affected areas.

❧ Insect bite, venereal diseases : Boil the following in 1 cup water: $1/2$ tsp each cynodon roots, cumin, liquorice, galangal and pomegranate flowers. Take twice daily for a few days.

❧ Itch, psoriasis, ringworm, rashes : Grind equal quantities of the following along with the required amount of buttermilk into a fine paste: bermuda grass, rind of chebulic myrobalan, rock salt, *kanjaankorai*. Apply the paste on the affected areas of the skin.

❧ Nosebleeds : Extract the pure sap of the cleaned grass and use as nasal drops. (*Caution:* Take all precautions to prevent infection.)

❧ Obesity : Mix the juices of cynodon and carrot (1:1) and drink every morning for a month.

❧ Prickly heat : Grind a handful of grass blades into a very fine paste. Apply over the affected areas.

❧ Sexual debility : Grind the tender grass into a paste. Boil 1 tsp in 1 cup cow's milk along with the required quantity of sugar and take at bedtime every day for a month.

❧ Toxins in the body due to over-medication, pain due to gonorrhoea, piles, urinary discharge with pain, urine retention : Boil 1 tsp cleaned roots of eynodon along with $1/8$ tsp white pepper in a glass of water. Add $1/8$ tsp white butter to it and drink.

♣ To tone up flabby muscles, to sharpen the intellect and to impart brightness and facial beauty	: Grind 2 tbsp cleaned grass along with the root into a fine paste. Mix in an equal quantity of white butter. Eat twice a day for 45 days.
♣ Whitlow	: Apply the paste of the cleaned grass externally.
♣ Wounds	: Extract the juice from the leaves and apply on the wounds.
♣ Wounds and injuries	: Grind equal quantities of the cleaned grass with *bariara* (prickly sida) into a fine paste and apply on the wounds.

Note: Individual results may vary.

A Word of Caution

It is often advised that the joints of durva grass be removed before using it for medicinal purposes. Washing the grass in running water is also necessary to remove soil-particles and germs, particularly when its sap is to be used as eye drops, etc. Any carelessness on the part of the patient would lead to a situation where durva grass instead of eliminating an infection may end up causing yet another!

Oil

Moothanda Maamuni Tailam is a forbiddingly long Tamil name for a very simple but effective massage oil for the head.

The oil can be prepared quite easily with just a few ingredients available at any grocer's.

Clean durva with its roots well and cut into thin pieces. Tie loosely 4 tsp of these pieces with 4 tsp black pepper and 3 tsp cumin in a clean thin cloth and allow it soak in 1/2 litre gingelly oil, kept in a wide-mouthed earthen pot. Now tie the mouth of the pot tightly with another piece of cloth to prevent dust etc. from getting into it. Leave this pot out for 48 days under the sun. Don't forget to stir the oil every day while being careful not to disturb the cloth-pack of herbs inside.

After a month, the oil is fit for use. Massage the head well with this oil every day. Avoid using any other oil, hair-cream, shampoo or soap while using it. You can however rinse out your hair with plain water whenever you feel like.

Massaging the head every day with the oil for 40 to 80 days is supposed to improve deterorating eyesight. Besides, specific eye-related complaints such as myopia, cataract, night-blindness, etc. are also believed to be cured.

In Science

Aiyer, K. N. and M. Kolammal. 1963. *Pharmacognosy of Ayurvedic Drugs*. Trivandrum. (As a remedy for aggravated *kapha*, *pitta* and *rakta*.)

Bhatt, J. V. and R. Broker. 1953. Action of some plant extracts on pathogenic *Staphylococci*. *J. Sci. Industr. Res*. 12B: 540–542. (Antibiotic properties.)

Chopra, R. N. et al. 1956. *Glossary of Indian Medicinal Plants*. New Delhi: Council of Scientific and Industrial Research. 88. (Use in ophthalmia.)

Devsarmah, G. C. et al. 1986. Some doubtful medicinal plants of Assam with their identification and medicinal value. *Nagarjun* 29(10–12):1–4. (The plant paste applied on the wound helps in the immediate stoppage of bleeding; heals the wound if kept continuously bandaged for 3 consecutive days.)

Hartwell, J. L. 1969. Plants used against cancer—A survey. *Lloydia* 32(2):153–205. (Significant anti-cancer activity.)

Joshi, C. G. and N. G. Narar. 1952. Antibiotic activity of some Indian medicinal plants. *J. Sci. Industr. Res.* 11B(6):261. (Antibiotic activity documented.)

Karnıck, C. R. 1972. Some aspects of crude Indian drug plants used in Ayurvedic system of medicine for Madhumeha (Diabetes). *Acta Phytother. Amst.* 19(8):141–149. (Diuretic and hypoglycaemic activity noted.)

Masilamani, G. et al. 1981. Study of *karappan* (Eczema). *J. Res. Ayur. Siddha* 2(2):109–121. (Brings eczema under control.)

Odenigbo, G. O. and P. I. Awachie. 1993. Anti-convulsant activity of aqueous ethanolic extract of *Cynodon dactylon. Filoterapia* 64(5):447–449.

Rai, M. K. 1985. Plants used as medicine by the tribes of Chhindwara District, Madhya Pradesh. *J. Econ. Taxon. Bot.* 7(2):385–387. (Treatment for impotency.)

Sairam, T. V. 1998. Cynodon. *Dignity Dialogue*, March 27–28.

Singh, R. N. 1971. Screening of plant extracts and their isolates' fungicidal value. *Zabdeu J. Sci. Tech.* 9B(2):136–137. (Antifungal properties noted.)

Subramanian, S. et al. 1986. Wound-healing properties of *Cynodon dactylon* and *Pongamia glabra.* (Abstract of papers.) *Indian J. Pharmacol.* 18(1):47.

20

Carrot

Daucus carota

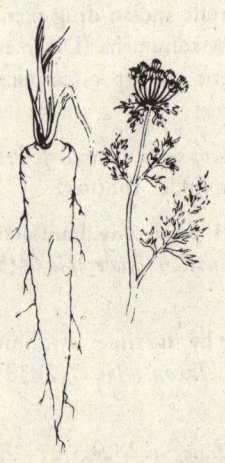

Useful in vitiated conditions of pitta . . .

—Dhanvantari Nighantu

Carrots and the Greeks

Archaeologists have unearthed yet another fact: the ancient Greeks cultivated carrots. In Greek, the intimacy between close friends was often referred to as that 'between the horse and the carrot'.

The carrot is not a native of India. It appears to have been introduced into India from Afghanistan in the remote past.

It is however a popular tuber in Indian cuisine, both raw and cooked. Besides starch, sugar, iron, calcium and phosphorous, it contains appreciable amounts of Vitamins—A, B and C. The wild carrot, whose seeds are used medicinally, has tough, white, inedible roots.

Food for Emperors

The *Ain-e-Akbari* written during Akbar's time notes that the leaves and roots of the carrot were included in the daily diet of the Emperor. Abul Fazl, the author, has also described in mouth-watering detail the tangy carrot pickle which no doubt titillated the tastebuds of the Emperor.

Medicinal Use of the Carrot

A diuretic, stimulant, carminative, anthelmintic, emmenagogue and aphrodisiac, the carrot has many a medicinal use, particularly in deficiency diseases. The carrot's appreciable level of potassium salts accounts for its diuretic action, and an essential oil for its onslaught on roundworms. It is also useful in preventing putrefaction in the intestine and in gastrointestinal catarrh.

Raw carrots have been shown to depress blood cholesterol. In one study, consumption of about 200 gm raw carrot a day (about 2 to 3 medium-sized carrots) brought down blood cholesterol at an average of 11 per cent.

Profile

Botanical Name	:	*Daucus carota* L. var. *sativa* DC.
English Names	:	Bee's Nest, Carrot, Wild Carrot.
Indian Names	:	Hindi : *Gajar, Gajra*
		Kannada : *Gajjari*
		Malayalam : *Kaarattu, Munna Mullangi*
		Sanskrit : *Gajarah*
		Tamil : *Manjal Mullangi, Gajjara Kilangu*
		Telugu : *Gajaragade.*

Family	:	Umbelliferae.
Appearance	:	An annual or biennial herb. Stem, hairy and branched. Leaves, in fine divisions. Flowers, lacy, white, in clusters.
Distribution	:	Cultivated chiefly in Punjab, Uttar Pradesh and Madhya Pradesh.
Medicinal Parts	:	Root (cultivated), leaves and seeds (wild).
Preparation and Dose	:	*Infusion/decoction*: 1 tbsp seeds with 1 cup water. *Juice* : 1 to 2 cups a day. *Soup* : 1/2 kg peeled grated carrots boiled in 4 cups water.

In Tradition

AILMENT	PRESCRIPTION
♣ Amenorrhoea	: Boil 2 tsp seeds in a glass of water and strain. Add 1 tsp jaggery and drink every day for a week.
♣ Anaemia	: Mix 2 tbsp each honey and the juice of carrot and drink for a few days.
♣ Anaemia, blood impurities, diabetes, eczema, threadworm infection, urine retention	: Frequent intake of carrot juice.
♣ Arthritis, blood impurities, pain in joints, ulcers	: The leaves are to be included in the daily diet.

❧ Cataract	: Take carrot and onion juice mixed with some yoghurt (1/3 cup each) with 1/4 tsp powdered pepper every morning. (*Note:* This is a preventive measure.)
❧ Cholesterol, roundworm infection	: 2–3 raw carrots a day for several days.
❧ Diarrhoea, intestinal disorders	: Hot carrot soup will soothe and quicken the natural healing process.
❧ Glaucoma	: Mix equal quantities of the juices of carrot and cynodon and drink once a day.
❧ Gum diseases, gum inflammation, mouth-ulcer	: Chew the raw leaves 2 or 3 times a day and wash the mouth out.
❧ Hair loss	: Take a glassful of a mixture of carrot, alfalfa and lettuce juices.
❧ Obesity	: Take a glass of carrot juice along with powdered black peppercorns (10) every morning.
❧ Palpitation of the heart	: Bury some carrots in hot ashes. When tender, slice and place in the open overnight in a ceramic dish to catch the dew. In the morning, sprinkle some sugar and rose water over them, and eat for a few days.

Note: Individual results may vary.

In Science

Agarwal, S. L. 1953. Chemical and pharmacological investigations of seeds of *Daucus carota*. *Indian Pharmacist* 8:291. (Blood pressure brought down by the seeds.)

Bhargava, A. K. et al. 1967. Pharmacological investigation of essential oil of *Daucus carota*. *Indian J. Pharm.* 29(4):127. (Cardiac depressant effect.)

Carper, Jean. 1989. *The Food Pharmacy—Damatic New Evidence that Food is Your Best Medicine*. Simon & Schuster. 156–159.

Chaudhury, R. R. and M. Haq. 1980. Review of plants screened for anti-fertility activity. *Bull. Medico-Ethno-Bot. Res.* 1(3)408. (A post-coital contraceptive agent.)

Chopra, R. N. et al. 1956. *Glossary of Indian Medicinal Plants*. New Delhi: Council of Scientific and Industrial Research. 91. (Relieves uterine pain.)

Colditz, G. A. et al. 1987. Diet and Lung Cancer—A review of the epidemiologic evidence in humans. *Archives of Internal Med.* 147:157–160.

Dhar, U. J. et al. 1975. Pharmacological studies on *Daucus carota*. *Planta Med.* 28(1):12. (Abortifacient.)

Gambhir, S. S. et al. 1966. Studies on *Daucus carota* Linn. Part I. Pharmacological studies with the water-soluble fraction of the alcoholic extract of the seeds—a preliminary report. *Indian J. Med. Res.* 54:178. (Relaxes the smooth muscles.)

_____.1966. Studies on *Daucus carota* Linn. Part II. Cholinergic activity of the quaternary-base isolated from water-soluble fraction of seeds. *Indian J. Med. Res.* 54:1053.

_____.1968. Pharmacological studies of tertiary base from seeds of *Daucus carota*. *Indian J. Physiol. Pharmacol.* 12:35. (Relaxant.)

_____.1979. Antispasmodic activity of tertiary base of *Daucus carota* seeds. *Indian J. Physiol. Pharmacol.* 23(3):225.

Garg, R. P. et al. 1973. Antiprogestational activity of seeds of *Daucus carota* in rats. *Indian J. Pharmac.* 5:282.

Garg, S. K. 1973. Anti-fertility effect and mechanism of action of chromatographic fractions of *Daucus carota* Linn. (seeds). *Indian J. Pharmac.* 5:272.

Garg, S. K. and G. P. Garg. 1970. Anti-fertility screening of plants. Part VII. Effect of five indigenous plants on early pregnancy of albino rats. *Indian J. Med. Res.* 59:302. (Abortifacient.)

_____. 1978. Screening of Indian plants for anti-fertility. *Indian J. Exptl. Biol.* 16(10):1077.

Gupta, S. P. et al. 1972. Pharmacological screening of seeds of *Daucus carota* Linn. with special reference to their anti-fertility activity. *Indian J. Pharmac.* 4:101

Kapoor, M. et al. 1974. Anti-ovulatory activity of five indigenous plants in rabbits. *Indian J. Med. Res.* 62(8):1225.

Lal, Ramesh. et al. 1986. Anti-fertility effect of *Daucus carota* seeds in female albino rats. *Filoterapia* 57(4):243.

Meena, S. et al. 1986. Anti-microbial activity of the essential oils of Umbelliferae. Part II. *Pak. J. Sci. Industr. Res.* 29(3):189. (Fights micro-organisms.)

Menkes, M. S. et al. 1986. Serum-beta carotene, vitamins A and E. Selenium and the risk of lung cancer. *New England J. of Med.* 315(20):1250–1254. (Individuals with the lowest blood levels of beta-carotene compared with those with the most were four times more likely a decade later to develop squamous cell carcinoma of the lung, the most common cancer due to cigarette smoking.)

Norell, S. E. et al. 1986. Diet and Pancreatic Cancer—A case-control study. *American J. Epidemiol.* 124(6):894–902

Peto, R. et al. 1981. Can dietary B-carotene materially reduce human cancer rates? *Nature* 290:210–208.

Rafi Khan. 1977. Anti-fertility activity of the seeds of *Daucus carota*. *Nagarjun* 21(4):8.

147

Robertson, J. et al. 1979. The effect of raw carrot on serum lipids and colon function. *American J. Clin. Nutr.* 32(9):1889–1892.

Shekelle, R. B. et al. 1981. Dietary Vitamin A and risk of cancer in the Western Electric study. *Lancet* 1185–1189. (Male smokers, even those who had smoked for 30 years, who ate the least beta-carotene containing foods had eight times the risk of developing lung cancer as those who ate the most beta-carotene containing foods, mainly carrots.)

Udupa, K. N. and R. H. Singh. 1979. Anti-fertility property of the alcoholic extract of carrot seed. *J. Res. Indian Med. Yoga and Homoeo.* 14(1):128.

Ziegler, R. G. et al. 1986. Carotenoid intake, vegetables and the risk of lung cancer among white men in New Jersey. *American J. Epidemiol.* 123(6):1080–1093. (Men who ate a mere half-cup of carrots a day were half as likely to develop lung cancer as those who ate almost none. In addition to carrots the other two vegetables which stood out in preventing lung cancer were: sweet potatoes and dark yellow winter squash.)

21

Jamun

Eugenia jambolana

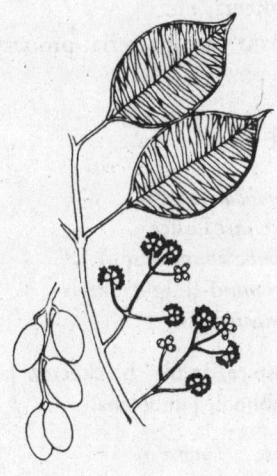

*In the continent where
jambu grows
And where the land of
Bharata lies . . .*

—Hindu Ritual Invocation

Wine, Vinegar and Medicine

The jamun in Hindu mythology is associated with the elephant-headed Ganesha and Lord Krishna. It is also sacred to the Buddhists. The ripe fruit of the jamun tree is eaten widely in India. A wine is prepared from the pulp in Goa. The juice of the unripe fruit is used in the preparation of a vinegar. The blossoms are an important source of honey.

There are two major varieties of jamun, one bearing large fruits and the other with smaller but fleshier fruits. Both have varied medicinal uses, apart from having delighted centuries of truant children. Jamun seeds find their popular use in the treatment of diabetes in India. They are also known for their CNS-depressant activity. Their hypoglycaemic and CNS-depressant roles have been confirmed in various laboratory experiments carried out at the Central Drug Research Institute, Lucknow. Extracts of leaves and bark apart from the seeds are also used in the treatment of diabetes.

The jamun's bark is astringent and used to treat asthma, bronchitis, dysentery, sore throat, ulcers, etc.

Science has also endorsed the plant's antibacterial properties.

Profile

Botanical Names	:	*Eugenia jambolana* Lam. *Engenia cuminii* Druce *Eugenia jambolanum* (Lam.) DC *Syzigium cuminii* (Linn.) Skeels *Myrtus cuminii* Linn.
English Names	:	Indian Allspice, Indian Blackberry, Java Plum, Jambhool, Jambolana.
Indian Names	:	Andamanese : *Thabye* Assamese : *Jamu* Bengali : *Jam, Kalojam* Gujarati : *Jambu, Jamli* Hindi : *Jamun, Jambu, Jambava Phalendra* Lepcha : *Phoberkung* Malayalam : *Yavel* Marathi : *Jambhul, Jamun* Nepali : *Kalajam* Oriya : *Jamkuk, Jamo* Punjabi : *Jammu* Sanskrit : *Jambu, Phalendra* Tamil : *Nagapazham, Naval* Telugu : *Neredu.*

Family	:	Myrtaceae.
Appearance	:	A large evergreen tree with light grey bark and dark grey patches; leaves, smooth and oval, in pairs; flowers, small, numerous, sweet scented, dull-white in bunches; fruit, dark purplish-black, juicy when ripe; seeds, round and smooth.
Distribution	:	Cultivated throughout India, generally along riverbanks and in wet places. Also distributed over Australia, Malaysia and Sri Lanka.
Medicinal Parts	:	Bark, fruit, kernel, leaves, seeds.
Ayurvedic Preparations	:	*Lohasinduram, Varahyadighrtam, Usirasavam.*
Other Uses	:	Seeds used as fodder too.

In Tradition

AILMENT	PRESCRIPTION
❧ Bad breath, blood in stools, dysentery	: Powder the bark and bottle. *Dose:* To 1 tsp powder, add 1 teacup warm water. Stir well. Gargle 4 to 5 times a day.
	: Deseed the fruit to obtain $1/2$ cup fruit pulp. Add an equal amount of sugar and heat the mixture over a low flame till it achieves a jam-like consistency. Now take off the fire and bottle. *Dose:* 1 tsp jam in 1 cup hot water twice daily.

❧ Burning sensation   : Eat 5 fruits every morning for a
during urination,   few days.
painful urination

❧ Burning sensation   : Eat 5 to 10 jamun fruits after breakfast
in eyes, early stages   every day.
of diabetes, watery
eyes

❧ Diabetes   : Powder the seeds and bottle. *Dose:* To
$1/4$ tsp of this powder, add 1 tsp honey
and take every morning for 45 days.

❧ Diarrhoea   : Grind the bark and extract 1 tbsp juice.
Add 1 tbsp goat's milk and stir well.
Drink.

❧ Diarrhoea,   : Extract 2 tsp juice from the tender
indigestion   leaves and buds. Add 1 tsp honey. Stir
well and drink.

❧ Dysentery   : Grind jamun fruits and mango
leaf-buds, a handful each, into a very
fine paste. Dilute with 1 cup buttermilk
and drink.

❧ Menorrhagia   : Boil in 2 teacups of water 2 tbsp finely
ground bark, till the volume is reduced
to 1 cup. *Dose:* 1 to 2 tbsp twice a day.

Note: Individual results may vary.

A Word of Caution

Continuous intake of jamun fruits may cause irritation of the throat.

In Science

Brahmachari, H. D. and K. T. Augusti. 1961. Hypoglycaemic agents from indigenous plants. London: *J. Pharm.* 13(6):381–382. (Fights diabetes.)

———— 1962. Orally effective hypoglycaemic agents from plants. London: *J. Pharm.* 14(4):254–255.

Chopra, R. N. et al. 1956. *Glossary of Indian Medicinal Plants.* New Delhi: Council of Scientific and Industrial Research. (The bark fights diarrhoea and the seeds, diabetes.)

Jain, S. R. and S. N. Sharma. 1967. Hypoglycaemic drugs of indigenous origin. *Planta Med.* 15(4):439–442.

Lal, B. N. and K. D. Chaudhuri. 1968. Observation on *Momordica charantia* (Karvellaka) and *Eugenia jambolana* (Jamboo) as oral antidiabetic remedies. *J. Res. Indian Med.* 2(2):161–164.

Maiti, A. P. et al. 1985. Comparison of minimum inhibitory concentration of water-soluble extracts of *Eugenia jambolana* bark of different ages on dysentery and diarrhoea forming micro-organisms. *Ancient Sci. Life* 5(2):113–115. (Water extracts of 10-year old bark exhibited antibacterial property against *S. dysenterae* and *S. boydi*.)

Mukherjee, B. 1957. Indigenous Indian drugs used in the treatment of diabetes. *J. Sci. Industr. Res.* 16A(10) (Suppl.):1–18.

————, 1962. Drug research—oral antidiabetic drugs. *East Pharm.* 5(49):35–43.

Nair, A. G. R. and S. Sankara Subramanian. 1962. Chemical examination of the flowers of *Eugenia Jambolana*. *J. Sci. Industr. Res.* 21B:457–458.

Nanda, C. V. et al. 1983. Effect of Jambu fruit pulp (*Eugenia jambolana* Lam.) on blood-sugar levels in healthy volunteers and diabetics. *J. Res. Ayur. Sid.* IV, 1–4:1–5. (Jambu fruit pulp does not exhibit any significant role in the management of diabetes.)

Shrotri, D. S. 1963. et al. Investigations of the hypoglycaemic properties of *Eugenia jambolana Indiah.. J. Med. Res.* 51(5):464–467. (Fruit juice administered orally to fasting rabbits produced 20–50% rise in blood-sugar in 2 hours. Afterwards, there was a steep fall of blood-sugar to a level below the fasting blood-sugar level. This could be due to higher sugar-content of the fruit. However, seeds exhibited significant hypoglycaemic effect, upto 20–23%.)

Sivarajan, V. V. and I. Balachandran. 1994. *Ayurvedic Drugs and their Plant Sources.* Madras: Oxford & IBH. p. 188.

Slowing, K. et al. 1994. Anti-inflammatory activity of *Eugenia jambolana* leaf extracts in rats. *J. Ethnopharmacol.* 43(1):9–11.

Sukh Dev. 1983. Natural products in medicine—present status and future prospects. *Curr. Sci.* 52(20):947–956.

Upadhyaya, V. P. 1984. Diabetes mellitus and its management by indigenous resources. *Nagarjun* 28(1 and 2):6–8.

22

Banyan

Ficus benghalensis

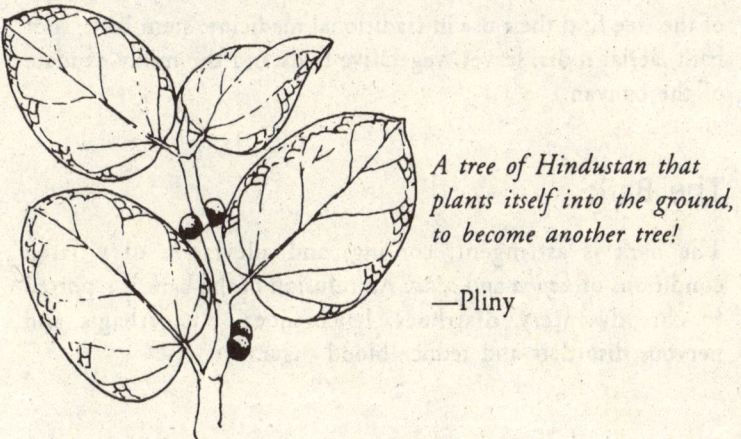

A tree of Hindustan that plants itself into the ground, to become another tree!

—Pliny

Tree of Mythic Proportions

It is no wonder that accounts of the banyan tend to speak with a tree with its trunk larger than four metres in girth, whose canopy spreads over fifty feet and with over a thousand aerial branches as in Sibpur, Calcutta! Or a tree said to be five hundred and odd years old, covering over three acres of landmass, as in Chunchunakuppe, Bangalore! And a tree that is circumambulated by women who seek to bear children! Small wonder then, that the ancient tourists of Hindustan were tempted to add the banyan to the list of several wonders they must have encountered here.

The Milk-Bearing Tree

The banyan is quite a common sight in the plains of India, providing much-needed relief from the hot Indian sun. The Britishers who found Hindu banias transacting their business briskly under the shade of this tree began to refer to it as the 'banyan'. It is one of the four great *Kshiravrikshas*, i.e. milk-exuding trees, the other three being *peepul (Ficus religiosa)*, *plaksa (Ficus lacor)* and *udumbara (Ficus glomerata)*. Several parts of the tree find their use in traditional medicine: stem bark, root bark, aerial roots, leaves, vegetative buds and the milky exudate of the banyan.

The Bark

The bark is astringent, cooling, and alleviative of vitiated conditions of *kapha* and *pitta*. An infusion of the bark is reported to cure dysentery, diarrhoea, leucorrhoea, menorrhagia and nervous disorders and reduce blood sugar.

The Leaves

A paste of the leaves is applied externally to abcesses and boils to promote suppuration.

The Aerial Roots

Tender aerial roots are chewed and used as toothbrushes. They are known to strengthen the gums and teeth. A paste of the tender twigs taken with cow's milk is reported to enhance sperm production. The fruits of this tree are also eaten for the same purpose.

Profile

Botanical Names	:	*Ficus benghalensis* L. *Urostigma benghalense* (L.) Gasp.
English Name	:	Banyan Tree.
Indian Names	:	Bengali : *Bot* Gujarati & Marathi : *Vad* Hindi : *Bar, Bargad,* *Nyagrodh* Kannada : *Ala* Malayalam : *Peral, Vatavriksham* Sanskrit : *Vatah* Tamil : *Aalamaram* Telugu : *Peddamari.*
Family	:	Moraceae.
Appearance	:	A large tree with aerial roots. Leaves, large and oval, deep green above and pale green beneath. Figs 1 or 2, axillary.
Distribution	:	Commonly found throughout the country from sea-level to an elevation of about 1000 m.
Medicinal Parts	:	Stem bark, root bark, aerial roots, leaves, vegetative buds, sap (milky exudate), flowers, fruits.
Ayurvedic Preparations:		*Chandanasavam, Dinesavalyadi Kulambu, Khadira Gulika, Kumkumadi Tailam, Saribadyasavam, Valiya Chandanadi Tailam,* etc.

In Tradition

AILMENT	PRESCRIPTION
❧ Abcess, boils	: Warm banyan leaves after coating them with gingelly oil and make a hot poultice to promote suppuration and hasten their breaking.
❧ Bad breath, gum problems, loosening teeth	: Mix the sap with honey and apply on the gums. Leave on for 10 minutes. Gargle.
❧ Bad breath, ulceration in mouth	: Boil 1 inch bark in 1 cup water for 5 minutes. Cool and use for gargling. Repeat 3 to 4 times a day.
❧ Bleeding piles	: A few drops of the sap of the tree to be taken in a glass of milk daily. Along with this treatment, add to the daily diet greens like fenugreek leaves, Black Nightshade (*manathakkali*) leaves, etc.
❧ Bruises, cracks on the sole, haemorrhoids, swelling	: Apply the latex externally.
❧ Conjunctivitis, gritty feeling in eyes, ophthalmia	: Grind together one clove and the sticky juice of the banyan tree into a very fine paste. Wrap in a clean muslin. Squeeze the drops into the eyes. (*Note:* 1. Take the necessary hygiene precautions to prevent infection. 2. This may cause irritation in the eyes.)
❧ Cracks in the heels	: Fill the cracks with the milk of the banyan tree.

❧ Diabetes

: Soak 1 inch bark overnight in a glass of water and drink the infusion the next morning.

: Boil 1 tbsp powdered bark in 2 cups water till the volume is reduced to $1/2$ cup. Filter and drink.

: Soak 1 tbsp chips of the bark overnight in a glass of water. Drink the infusion the next morning.

❧ Diarrhoea

: Soak the tender leaf-buds overnight in a glass of water. Drink the infusion the next morning.

: Soak 1 tsp powder of dried leaf-buds in a glass of water overnight. Next morning, drink the infusion. Fill the navel with the sap of the banyan tree.

❧ Eczema

: Char the tender leaf-buds in hot ashes. The ashes of the buds so obtained are dissolved in gingelly oil for application on the affected areas.

: Make a fine paste of the required amount of prop-roots in a little cow's urine and apply on the affected areas.

❧ Excessive urination

: Boil 2 tsp bark in 1 glass water till it is reduced to $1/2$ glass. Drink 1 tsp of the decoction twice or thrice a day.

❧ Female sterility

: Dry the tender roots of the banyan tree in the shade and make a fine powder. Take $1/2$ tsp of this powder along with milk (1 cup) for three consecutive nights after the menstruation cycle ends every month, till conception occurs. (*Note:* While undergoing this treatment, no other food should be taken in the night.)

❦ Gum problems, pyorrhoea

: Clean the mouth with the aerial roots: chew the crushed aerial roots and wash the mouth with lukewarm water.

: Boil $1/2$ tbsp bark in 2 cups water till the volume is reduced to $1/2$ cup. Add 1 tsp honey and drink for 90 days.

❦ Leucorrhoea

: Boil 1 tbsp each of the powdered bark from the fig tree and the banyan tree in 1 litre water till reduced to $1/2$ litre. Strain and when lukewarm, douche the vagina. Repeat 2 or 3 times a day.

: Boil 1 tbsp bark in 2 cups water till the volume is reduced to $1/2$ cup. Add $1/2$ cup milk and 1 tsp palmyrah sugar and drink. Once daily for 15 days.

❦ Lumbago, rheumatism

: Apply the sap of the banyan tree on the affected areas.

❦ Mouth-ulcer, ulceration on the tongue

: Apply a mixture of sap and honey locally.

❦ Painful joints

: Heat 3 tbsp gingelly oil. Add a paste made of 4 to 5 banyan leaves and 4 to 5 garlic pods. Remove from the fire when boiling and when lukewarm, add 1 tsp used kerosene and mix well. Apply this paste on the affected parts.

❧ Painful joints : Coat the leaves with a little gingelly oil, warm them over a flame and apply on the affected parts.

❧ Pimples : Apply a finely ground paste of the young aerial roots. Repeat.

❧ Premature ejaculation : Smear 4 to 5 drops of banyan latex on a piece of *batasha* (a sweetmeat available in all North Indian towns) and take before sunset.

❧ Premature ejaculation, watery sperm : Dry the tender leaf-shoots of the banyan tree in the shade and powder before mixing it with an equal quantity of jaggery. *Dose:* Take 1 tsp of this mixture every morning along with a glass of milk.

❧ Rashes : Apply a paste of the leaves on the affected areas.

❧ Sexual debility : Fry a small piece of asafoetida in ghee. Mix $1/2$ tsp milk of the banyan tree with it and take in the morning.

❧ Skin diseases, venereal diseases : Boil 4 tbsp bark in 4 cups water till the volume is reduced to 1 cup. Add 1 tsp honey and drink. (2 or 3 times a week.)

❧ Stomach complaints : Soak some aerial roots (after washing them well) in drinking water along with leaves of the bitter-orange or jamun tree. Use the water for drinking.

❧ Vomiting : Boil 1 tbsp crushed tender ends of the

aerial roots in a glass of water for 10 minutes. Strain and sip when bearably warm.

Note: Individual results may vary.

In Science

Aiyer, M. N. et al. 1957. *Pharmacognosy of Ayurvedic Drugs.* Nos. 4–9. Trivandrum. (Protects the gums and teeth.)

Atiane, A. et al. 1985. Folk medicinal uses of *Ficus benghalensis* L. and *Punica granatum* L. in northern Uttar Pradesh. *Bull. Med. Ethnobot. Res.* 6(1):42–46. (The prop roots are found to be useful in checking external as well as internal bleeding in cases of menorrhagia, ulcers, etc.)

Moos, N. S. 1976. *Single Drug Remedies.* Kottayam.

Nadkarni, A. K. 1954. *Indian Materia Medica.* Bombay. (Strengthens gums.)

Singh, N. et al. 1992. Study of anti-diabetic effect of alcoholic extracts of *Ficus benghalensis* Linn. on alloxan diabetic albino rats. *J. Res. Ayur. Siddha.* (Brings down blood pressure, serum cholesterol and blood-urea levels.)

Vinod Kumar, R. and K. T. Augusti. 1992. Anti-diabetic effect of a leucocyanidin derivative isolated from the bark of *Ficus benghalensis* Linn. *Indian J. Biochem. Biophys.* 26(6):400–404. (Lowers the fasting blood-glucose level.)

———. 1993. Insulin sparing action of a leucocynidin derivative isolated from *Ficus benghalensis* Linn. *Amala Res. Bull.* 13:32–36. (Useful in treating diabetes.)

23

Peepul

Ficus religiosa

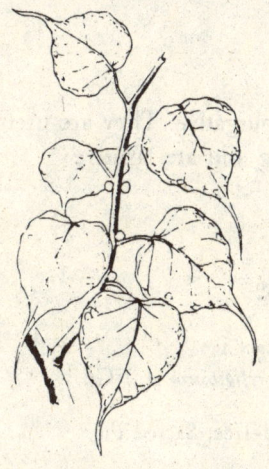

Among the trees, I am asvattha . . .

—Lord Krishna in the *Bhagavad Gita*

The Auspicious Tree

The peepul is one of the most sacred trees of the Hindus and is often planted in the vicinity of temples and holy places. The planting of the tree is considered an auspicious event of great importance to the planter, as generations to come will be benefited by this noble act. Like the tulsi, the peepul is also believed to possess supernatural powers.

For the Buddhists, the tree has immense symbolic value: it stands for knowledge and its awakening (*bodhi*).

The Peepul's Bark

The peepul's bark contains 4% tannin and is astringent. It forms an important ingredient in several Ayurvedic formulations. Its infusion is found to be effective in the treatment of ulcers and skin ailments. It alleviates *pitta* and *kapha* and improves the complexion. Bacteriologists have confirmed its antibacterial activity, especially against *Staphylococcus aureus* and *Escherichia coli*.

Leaf-Buds and Seeds

The leaves and tender shoots are purgative. They are useful in skin diseases. The seeds are cooling and are laxative.

Profile

Botanical Names	:	*Ficus religiosa* L.
		Urostigma religiosum (L.) Gr.
English Names	:	Peepul, Bo-Tree, Sacred Fig.
Indian Names	:	Bengali : *Asvattha*
		Gujarati : *Jari, Pipro, Pipul*
		Hindi : *Pipal*
		Kannada : *Arali, Aswattha*
		Malayalam : *Arasu, Arayal, Asvattham, Avasai*
		Marathi : *Ashwatha, Pimpala*
		Sanskrit : *Ashwatta, Bodhadruma, Pippala*
		Tamil : *Arasamaram*
		Telugu : *Aswatthamu, Bodhi, Raavi.*
Family	:	Moraceae.

164

Appearance	:	Large tree with characteristic milky exudate; deltoid papery leaves with very long petioles which produce rustling music at the slightest puff of wind. Bark is smooth and light grey in colour, peeling off in bits and patches. Flowers, inconspicuous and colourless. Fruits green and smooth when unripe; purple when ripe.
Distribution	:	Common in most parts of India. Also known in South East Asia.
Medicinal Parts	:	Bark, leaf-buds, seeds.
Ayurvedic Preparations	:	*Chandanasavam, Kachoradi Tailam, Karnasulantakam, Nalpamaradi Tailam, Saribadyasavam, Valiya Marmagulika.*

In Tradition

AILMENT	PRESCRIPTION
❦ Bleeding piles	: Take 1 tsp dried leaf powder with warm water.
❦ Boils, mumps, pustules	: Take a peepul leaf. Smear it with ghee and warm slightly over a naked flame. Use as bandage when lukewarm on the affected parts.
❦ Burns, swellings	: Apply a paste of the powdered bark locally.
❦ Complexion-improvement	: Mix bark powder and besan powder in equal quantities and use in place of soap for cleansing the face and hands.

♣ Constipation : Dry a few peepul leaves in the shade and powder them along with 1 tsp aniseed. Add a little jaggery and water and form into pills. Take 2–3 pills with warm milk before going to bed every day.

♣ Cracks in the sole : Chip off the bark and collect the latex (milk). Apply on the soles.

♣ Diabetes, nervous diseases : Soak some crushed bark in a glass of water overnight. Filter. Drink the filtrate in the early morning for a few days. (*Note:* This increases the urine output.)

♣ Diarrhoea : Mix 1 tsp each nutmeg powder and bark powder in a glass of buttermilk and drink 2–3 times.

♣ Earache : Boil some crushed bark pieces and mustard oil. Strain and use this oil as ear drops.

♣ Ear infection, otitis media : Extract the juice from the leaves. Warm slightly and pour 2–3 drops into the ear with the help of cotton wool.

♣ Female sterility : Fry a few tender leaf-buds in ghee. Eat them with a glass of milk during the menstrual period.

♣ Itch, skin diseases : Grind the bark into a fine powder and and bottle. Mix 1 tsp of this powder in a little coconut oil and apply on the affected areas.

- Lesions and wounds: Burn a few tender leaf-buds and mix
  in feet developed   the ash with some coconut oil. Apply
  due to moisture in   on the affected areas, in between
  tropical areas   fingers, toes, etc.

- Leucorrhoea,   : Soak some crushed bark overnight in
  menorrhagia,   a mug of water and use it to douche
  urino-genital   the affected areas frequently.
  disorders,
  vaginal diseases

- Leucorrhoea,   : Dry a few peepul fruits in the shade
  nocturnal emiss-   and powder them. Take $1/2$ to 1 tsp of
  ions, premature   this powder along with a glass
  ejaculation, sexual   of milk every night before going to bed
  debility,   for a few days.
  spermatorrhoea

- Scabies,   : Dry and grind the bark into a fine
  skin diseases   powder. Dust this bark on the affected
                         areas frequently.

- Soreness in the   : Apply the finely ground powder of the
  mouth   bark on the gums, tongue and inside
                         the mouth-wall frequently.

Note: Individual results may vary.

In Science

Benthall, A. P. 1946. *The Trees of Calcutta and its Neighbourhood.* Calcutta: Thacker, Spink & Co.

Chopra, R. N. 1933. *Indigenous Drugs of India: Their Medical and Economic Aspects.* Calcutta.

HOME REMEDIES

Kirtikar, K. R. and B. D. Basu. 1935. *Indian Medicinal Plants*. Allahabad. III:2318. (In the Indian systems of medicine.)

Nadkarni, K. M. 1927. *Indian Materia Medica*. Bombay. (Medicinal uses.)

Pearson, R. S. and H. P. Brown. 1932. *Commercial Timbers of India*. 2 Vols. Calcutta: Central Publication Branch. (Economic uses listed.)

Rama Rao, M. 1914. *Flowering Plants of Travancore*. Trivandrum: Government Press.

Sairam, T. V. Peepul. *Dignity Dialogue* 2(11): 31–36.

Troup, R. S. 1921. *The Sylviculture of Indian Trees*. 3 Vols. Oxford: Oxford University Press.

24

Kutaja

Holarrhena antidysenterica

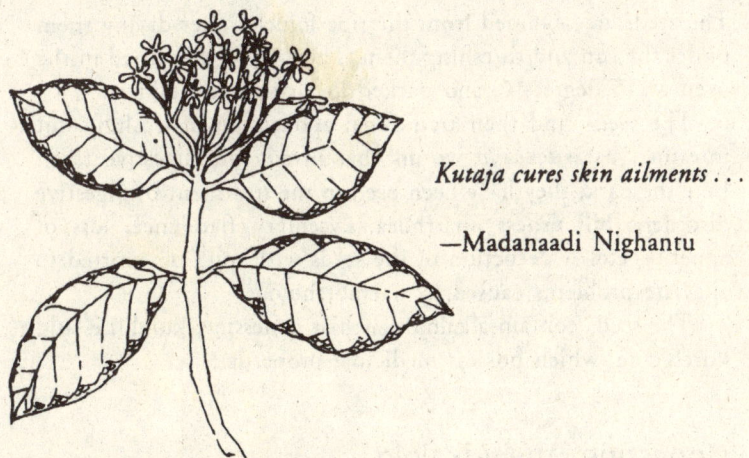

Kutaja cures skin ailments . . .

—Madanaadi Nighantu

Plant of the Peaks

Kutaja, the Sanskrit name of the plant, refers to its habitat: the peaks of mountainous terrain. The drug Kutaja consists of the dried stem bark collected from trees which are over 10 years old. As the bark is reported to contain a higher concentration of alkaloids immediately after the rains, the native physicians commence their collection during the post-monsoon months i.e., July to September.

In Ayurveda the drug is used in acute and chronic amoebic dysentery. Hence its botanical name *antidysenterica*. The drug is experimentally proved to be toxic to *Entamoeba histolytica*.

In folk medicine, a paste made of the dried bark is rubbed over the body in cases of dropsy. It is also traditionally used in the treatment of leprosy. It has tonic and febrifuge properties.

The alkaloids isolated from the bark include conessine, nor-conkurchicine and lettocine, which are the active substances.

The Seeds

The seeds are obtained from the ripe follicles after drying them under the sun and threshing them. They are further dried in the oven at 45 degrees C and packed in air-tight containers.

The seeds find their traditional application in flushing out intestinal parasites and worms that invade the digestive tract. Like the bark, they have been used in the treatment of digestive disorders: biliousness, diarrhoea, dysentery, flatulence, loss of appetite, etc. A decoction of the seeds with milk is reported to alleviate problems caused by haemorrhoids.

The seeds contain alkaloids such as conessine, kurchine, and kurchicine, which possess medicinal properties.

Conessine, the Alkaloid

The main alkaloidal constituent of the plant, conessine, is an established amoebicide. It kills dysentery bacilli *in vitro* and is also useful against cysts. It is also reported to raise the blood pressure in small doses; however, in larger doses it tends to be hypotensive. Conessine is said to be more effective than emetine and can be administered orally.

The leaves are also medicinally useful.

Environment-Friendly

Kutaja has a marked role in setting right ecological imbalances:

it has played a salient role in several afforestation programmes as a pioneer.

Profile

Botanical Names	:	*Holarrhena antidysenterica* (Linn.) Wall. ex. DC
		Holarrhena codaga G. Don.
		Holarrhena maloccensis Wight.
		Holarrhena pubescens (Buch.-Ham.) Wallich ex. Don.
		Echites antidysenterica Roxb.
		Wrightia antidysenterica Grah.
English Names	:	Conessi, Easter Tree, Kurchi, Talligherry, Tellicherry Tree.

Indian Names :

Assamese	: *Dutkhuri*
Bengali	: *Kurchi, Titaindarju*
Gujarati	: *Kuda*
Hindi	: *Dhudi, Indrajau, Indrajav, Indrayava, Karchi, Kari, Korai, Kura, Kurchi*
Kannada	: *Hale, Kodagasana, Korchu, Kudsalu*
Malayalam	: *Pala, Kodagapala, Panipalai, Venpala*
Marathi	: *Dudhari, Gal, Kodaya*
Oriya	: *Kherwa, Khurni*
Punjabi	: *Kewar*
Sanskrit	: *Girimallika, Kalinga, Kutaja*
Tamil	: *Erukalapalai, Indraban, Kalingam, Kasappuveppilai, Kirimalligai, Kudapalai, Kudasapalai, Pala, Vattagam, Veppalai*

171

Telugu	:	*Amkudu, Chedukodise, Giri Mallika, Istarakupala, Kalingamu, Kodaga, Kodisephala, Kutajamu, Pala Kodsa, Pala Berrai, Vistarakupala*
Naini Tal	:	*Keora*
Ayurvedic	:	*Kutaja*
Unani	:	*Kura, Teewaj.*

Family	:	Apocynaceae.
Appearance	:	Shrub or small tree with milky latex. Leaves, shiny above, dull and hairy below, with conspicuous nerves. Leaf-stalk very small. Flowers, white, in terminal bunches. Fruits, slender and paired, cylindrical, dark grey with white specks all over. Seeds, oblong with long tuft of hair.
Distribution	:	Throughout the drier parts, particularly in deciduous forests upto an altitude of 1000m. Also distributed in tropical Himalayas, Burma, Indo-China and Malaysia.
Medicinal Parts	:	Stem bark, root, seeds, leaves.
Dosage and Prescription	:	Bark: 1 to 1$^1/_2$ tsp of bark powder along with 1 tsp honey, twice a day. Seeds: $^1/_2$ to 1 tsp seed powder.
Ayurvedic Preparations	:	*Kutajghan Bati, Kutajavleh, Bismuth Kurchi.*
Unani Formulations	:	*Majoon-e-Teewaj, Majoon-e-Bawaseer, Suffof-e-Habis.*

In Tradition

AILMENT	PRESCRIPTION
✤ Amoebic dysentery, biliousness, flatulence	: Mix $1/4$ to $1/2$ tsp of the seed powder in warm water and drink.
✤ Blood in urine	: Grind half tsp each of the seeds of kutaja and vidanga. Add 1 cup water and drink.
✤ Cholera	: Mix $1/2$ tsp each of the powdered bark of siora and kutaja. Add 1 cup water and drink.
✤ Dropsy	: A paste made of the bark is rubbed on the body.
✤ Dysentery, loss of appetite	: Mix $1/4$ tsp bark powder in $1/2$ tsp honey and take.
✤ Haemorrhoids	: Boil $1/4$ tsp seed powder in milk and drink.

Note: Individual results may vary.

In Science

Anandakumar, A. et al. 1984. *Kutajabija*—its pharmacognosy. *Anc. Sci. Life* 3(4):203–206. (The medicinal properties of the seeds.)

Baksh, I. 1936. Pharmacological action of conessine and iso-conessine. *J. Pharmacol.* 58:373. (The alkaloid, conessine, obtained from the bark has been reported to retard the growth of Tubercle bacilli.)

Baksh, I. 1936. Action of kurchine, an alkaloid of *Holarrhena antidysenterica. J. Pharmacol.* 58:361.

Bertho, A. 1944. Pharmacological tests on the extracts and alkaloids of *Holarrhena antidysenterica. Arch. Exp. Path. Pharmacol.* 230:41.

Janot, M. M. et al. 1970. Steroid alkaloids. *Tetrahedron* 26:1695.

Khuong-Huu, Q. et al. 1971. Steroid alkaloids. CXIV. *Bull. Soc. Chim. Fr.* 3:864.

Manske, R. P. (ed.) *The Alkaloids: Chemistry and Physiology.* New York: Academic Press. Vol VI. p. 819; Vol. V. p. 312; Vol. IX. p. 320.

Roy, A. C. and B. Mukerji. 1958. Kurchi alkaloids: Thier isolation, constitution and biological activity. *J. Sci. Industr. Res.* 17A:158.

Satyavati, G. V. et al. Eds. 1987. *Medicinal Plants of India.* New Delhi.

Singh, K. P. 1986. Clinical studies on amoebiasis and giardiasis. Evaluating the efficacy of *kutaja (Holarrhena antidysenterica)* in *Entamoeba histolytica* cyst passers. *Anc. Sci. Life* 5(4):228–231. (Root bark found effective.)

25

Jasmine

Jasminum grandiflorum

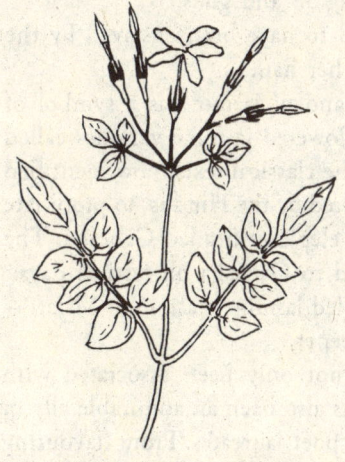

'Malati, the princess . . .'

—Abhidhana Manjari

Jasmine: The Chemistry of Sensuousness

The human nostrils contains bunches of highly sensitive, minute cells, which act as receptors of smell. Unlike other cells in the body, these cells regenerate every month. They react with specific aromatic molecules of essential oils to produce sensation. The receptors trigger electro-chemical impulses, which are transmitted to the limbic system—a portion of the brain which responds to pleasures, emotions and memories that linger. It is here that certain brain-affecting chemicals called neuro-chemicals are released.

Chemists have discovered that these neuro-chemicals influence the state of our health and mental well-being: serotonin relaxes you and calms your temper; enkephalin soothes your pain and makes you feel an exhilarated *joie de vivre;* endorphin induces sexual appetite.

Jasmine's divine scent can reach upto a radius of seventy metres and communicate its presence to one and all so very beautifully. Perhaps it is the scent that has resulted in jasmine being closely associated with religion and gods.

Historically, Cleopatra is said to have been enslaved by the scent of jasmine and used it in her hair.

Thai buddhists regard a garland of jasmine as a symbol of respect and regard. The yellow flowered jasmine varieties called Svarnajati or Hemapushpika in the classical texts, now identified as *Jasminum humile* Linn. are offered by the Hindus to propitiate particularly, Lord Shiva and the elephant-headed Ganesha. The leaves of jasmine are also offered to Ganesha on festival days.

In India, many a woman is called Jasmine, Yasmin or Malati— the names of this wonderful creeper.

Sweet-smelling jasmine has not only been associated with aesthetic and spiritual uses. It has also been an admirable ally of cooks and physicians apart from poet-laureates. From flavouring teas and desserts to eliminating inflammations and intestinal worms, jasmine has proved its versatility time and again.

Two species of jasmine viz., *Jasminum grandiflorum* and *Jasminum angustifolium* have been the source of the drug, which is known for its efficacy against chronic ulcers and skin diseases.

The flowers and leaves have been praised warmly for their aphrodisiac qualities.

Ancient Ayurvedic texts refer in addition to malati, to Gandhamalati or Madhumalati, which according to some botanists is *Aganosma dichotoma,* an altogether different genus of the family Apocynaceae. Whatever be the case, jasmine has continued to be the most widely recognized flower in the subcontinent.

Profile

Botanical Names	:	*Jasminum grandiflorum* Linn.	
		Jasminum angustifolium Vahl.	
English Names	:	Spanish Jasmine, Catalonian Jasmine, Common Jasmine, Jasmine.	
Indian Names	:	Hindi	: *Mogra, Jaati, Chameli*
		Kannada	: *Mallige*
		Malayalam	: *Picchakam, Mullapoovu*
		Sanskrit	: *Malati, Hrdaya-Gandha, Jaati*
		Tamil	: *Malligai, Jaadhi-Malligai, Pichchi, Kodimalligai*
		Telugu	: *Jaji, Malati*
Arabic Name	:	*Yasmin.*	
Family	:	Oleaceae.	
Appearance	:	Climbing shrub. Compound leaves with 7 to 9 leaflets. Flowers, sweet-scented, white, with a long tubular corolla.	
Distribution	:	Subtropical regions, above 5000 feet sea-level: North West Himalayas, coastal Andhra Pradesh, Western Ghats, Nilgiris, Palani hills, etc. Often cultivated in the plains.	
Medicinal Parts	:	Flowers, leaves, roots, oil.	
Medicinal Preparations	:	Infusion (Steep 1 to 2 tsp flowers in 1 cup water; take 1 cup a day), paste, powder, medicated oil.	
Ayurvedic Preparations	:	*Malatyadi Tailam, Jatyadi Tailam, Jatyadi Ghritam, Kalyanaka Ghritam, Aranyatulsyadi Oil*, etc.	

| Other species | : *Aganosma dichotoma* (Apocynaceae) |
| | *Jasminum humile* Linn. (Oleaceae). |

In Tradition

AILMENTS	PRESCRIPTION
❧ Earache	: Grind the leaves into a very fine paste. To 1 cup of the paste, add 1 cup gingelly oil. Boil till reduced to half of the original volume. Store in a clean bottle, when cool. Instil 2 drops in the ear.
❧ Halitosis	: Chew jasmine leaves as such or with dried rind of lime twice or thrice daily for a fortnight.
❧ Headache	: Soak a handful of fresh jasmine flowers in a small cup of water for at least 1 hour; add $1/4$ tsp salt into this water and stir well to dissolve. Instil 2–3 drops in the nostrils twice or thrice daily, as needed.
❧ Headache, eye trouble, skin ailments	: Apply the oil extracted from the flowers locally.
❧ Itching due to lice or dandruff	: Grind a handful of jasmine roots along with 1 tbsp calamus powder. Squeeze the juice of a lime fruit into it and use instead of shampoo.
❧ Migraine	: Grind a handful of leaves with 2 tbsp dried ginger and 2 tbsp milk. Heat the

mixture and apply on the forehead. Tie a napkin tightly around the head.

❦ Psoriasis, skin ailments
: Grind a handful of fresh flowers and apply the paste on the affected areas. (*Note:* This can be substituted for soap by people who are hypo-allergenic.)

❦ Sexual debility in men
: Grind the leaves into a fine paste and apply around the genitals. Use a napkin to make a tight loin-cloth. Leave on overnight. (*Note:* Instead of the leaf-paste, flowers as such can be used.)

❦ Skin diseases
: Mix equal quantities of the powders of jasmine root and calamus. Squeeze some lime juice into the mixture and apply on the affected parts.

❦ Suppurating wounds
: Apply the oil (See under Earache, above) externally.

❦ Swellings
: Grind a handful of flowers with very little water and apply on the affected areas.

❦ Swellings in throat
: Fry a handful of jasmine leaves in 1 tbsp gingelly oil and tie around the throat when bearably hot.

❦ To stop the secretion of milk in young mothers
: Tie a handful of jasmine flowers around the breasts. Leave on for a few hours. Repeat daily for a few days.

❦ Ulcers in mouth, gums, throat
: Chew a few leaflets for 10 minutes and rinse out the mouth in lukewarm water. Repeat frequently.

: Grind equal quantities of dried jasmine leaves, liquorice root, chebulic myrobalan and Indian Barberry *(Berberis aristata)* into a very fine powder. Mix in some honey and apply this paste frequently over the interior of the mouth—on the gums, throat, etc.

❧ Wounds : Apply the leaf-paste on the affected areas.

Note: Individual results may vary.

Jasmine: A Note on Aphrodisiac Oils and Plant Aromatics

There is a strange belief that an aphrodisiac oil should contain some of the elements of human sweat, urine, faeces or semen, the traditionally impure wastes of the body, or other decaying elements. Indole, the most common aphrodisiac ingredient found in the perfumes of moth-pollinated flowers such as jasmine, lilac, madonna lily, narcissus, tube rose, etc. is surprisingly a constituent of the odour of rotting flesh.

The oil of jasmine has a sensuously rich, intense, animal-like quality which serves as an 'emotional invigorator or tonifier'. Although jasmine is believed to be a powerful aphrodisiac, modern science is yet to prove or disprove such claims.

Ayurveda has, however, employed plant aromatics as a cure to several ailments—both mental and physical. Today in the West, aromatherapy has become a commonly accepted system of alternative medicine. Even health insurance schemes have come forward to underwrite such treatment!

It is also believed that men and women react differently to

different smells and this has fuelled the multi-billion dollar perfume industry in the U.S.A. and France. Men are supposed to prefer spicy, woody scents, while women choose floral fragrances. Jasmine has been considered an ideal perfume for women although in ancient India both men and women used it.

Jasmine Oil

To a cup of milk, add the following oils: 1 drop of bergamot, 2 drops of clary sage, 3 drops of jasmine and 4 drops of lavender. Add all these to warm bath water. This makes an ideal bath oil, whose aroma clears away anxiety and tension.

Jasmine Massage Oil

Take a cup of sweet almond oil and mix into it 10 to 15 drops of the essential oil of jasmine. This is a dependable massage oil for the mentally depressed.

In Science

Chopra, R. N. et al. 1956. *Glossary of Indian Medicinal Plants.* New Delhi. p. 143.

Chunekar, K. C. 1982. *Bhavaprakasanighantu of Sri Bhavamisra, Commentary.* Varanasi. (In Hindi) (Jasmine as medicine.)

Kapoor, S. L. and R. Mitra. 1979. *Herbal Drugs in Indian Pharmaceutical Industry.* Lucknow. p. 71. (Malati and its varieties.)

Kirtikar, K. R. and B. D. Basu. 1918. *Indian Medicinal Plants.* Allahabad. p. 764–765.

Nadkarni, A. K. 1954. *Indian Materia Medica.* Bombay. p. 702.

Sharma, P. V. 1983. *Dravyaguna Vijnana.* Varanasi. p. 178. (In Hindi)

(*Jasminum angustifolium* can also be an alternative source of the drug, in addition to *Jasminum grandiflorum*.)

Singh, T. B. and K. C. Chunekar. 1972. *Glossary of Vegetable Drugs in Brhttrayi*. Varanasi. p. 307.

26

Henna

Lawsonia inermis

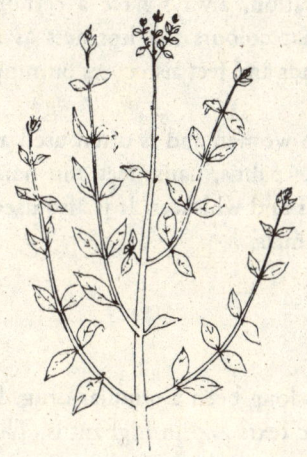

*Henna drives away
fevers . . .*

—Nighantu Ratnakaram

In Mythology

Henna is considered to be a herb sanctified by divine grace, and so believed to drive away evil spirits and their unhealthy influences. The dried fruits of this plant are considered to be the abode of Lakshmi, the Goddess of Wealth and Prosperity. In rural households, the fruits are plucked along with a bunch of leaves and are tied to the ceilings to ensure Lakshmi's presence.

Henna is also associated with Lord Shani (Saturn), who is one of the nine planets worshipped by the Hindus. When the malefic effects of Shani are feared, his devotees circumambulate the henna bush on Saturdays in order to appease his wrath and fury.

Ayurvedic Cosmetics

Ayurveda does not distinguish between food and medicine. The same concept is applied to the question of cosmetics as well. Cosmetics, though used for decoration, always have a certain medicinal value: tambool (pan) that colours the lips acts as a digestive; henna that colours the hands and feet also cures burning sensations in the limbs, kibes, etc.

Henna is also very popular with women and is often used as a fragrant orange dye to colour the palms, nails, feet and hair. Some men use it to dye their beards and whiskers. It is also used to dye the tails and fur of pet animals.

As Popular Medicine

In indigenous medicine, henna has long been a popular drug. It finds mention in ancient Ayurvedic texts and in nighantus. The *Shaligram Nighantu* speaks of the versatility of this drug. Its use in leprosy finds mention in the *Aswarishta Vijnan*. Its role as a blood purifier is recognized in the *Ayurveda Sarasangraha*.

Charaka and Sushruta have also studied this plant. *Mahaneelaghrita,* which is an important medicine used to treat several serious skin ailments such as leprosy, leucoderma, etc. contains henna as an important ingredient.

The leaves have certain medicinal properties: they are astringent and are used as a prophylactic against skin ailments. They are reported to be useful in haemorrhagia, tuberculosis and typhoid fever. However, pharmacological or clinical findings are lacking in this regard.

The flowers of henna yield an oil which finds its use in

perfumery. The seeds are reported to be an effective pesticide when powdered and soaked in water and sprayed on pest-infested trees.

Love-Potion

It is believed, in addition, that henna excites the passion of love.

Profile

Botanical Names	: *Lawsonia inermis* L. *Lawsonia alba* Lamk.	
English Names	: Henna, Egyptian Privet, Cypress Shrub, Indian Privet.	
Indian Names	: Bengali, Hindi, Gujarati Marathi & Punjabi	: *Henna, Mehndi*
	Kannada	: *Goranti, Madurangi, Mairanchi*
	Kashmiri	: *Mohuz*
	Malayalam	: *Mailanchi*
	Marathi	: *Mendhi*
	Oriya	: *Benjati*
	Punjabi	: *Hina*
	Sanskrit	: *Madayantika, Medhini, Mendika, Nakharanjani, Raktagarbha, Ragangi*
	Tamil	: *Azhavanam, Charanam, Eivanam, Marudhaani, Maruthondri, Mayilenandi, Niraththaan*
	Telugu	: *Goranta, Mullugorantla.*
Arabic Names	: *Al Khanna, Henna.*	

Family	:	Lythraceae.
Appearance	:	A shrub or a small tree, with branches 4-angled, usually ending in a sharp point. Leaves, green, also often with a sharp point. Flowers, small, sweet-smelling, white or pinkish, in large bunches. Fruit, round, pea-sized with many seeds.
Distribution	:	A native of Arabia and Persia, now cultivated throughout India as a hedge-plant. Commercial cultivation in the states of Gujarat, Madhya Pradesh, Punjab and Rajasthan.
Medicinal Parts	:	Bark, flowers, leaves, seeds.

In Tradition

AILMENT	PRESCRIPTION
❧ Boils, bruises, burns, leprosy	: Apply henna leaf-paste (early stages).
❧ Burning sensation in body	: Frequent local application of the oil expelled from the seeds.
❧ Burning sensation in feet	: Apply the crushed leaves on the soles of the feet and bandage.
❧ Burning sensation in feet, cracks	: Grind a handful of leaves into a fine paste. Mix in the juice of 1 lime. Apply on the affected parts at bedtime.
❧ Burning sensation in feet, headache	: Apply the leaf-paste on the affected parts.
	: Grind a handful of leaves with 1 tbsp lime juice and apply on the affected parts.

❦ Burns, syphilis   : Use an infusion of leaves for cleansing.

❦ Corns   : Grind a handful of henna leaves into a very fine paste along with 1 tsp each turmeric and calamus. Apply this paste on the affected areas at bedtime and tie a warmed betel leaf over it. The treatment should be continued for 21 days.

     : Grind the roots of the henna plant into a fine paste and apply on the affected areas for 40 days.

❦ Excessive urination : Grind henna leaves into a very fine paste. Take 1 tsp with a cup of cow's milk for a few days.

❦ Hair loss   : Boil 2 cups gingelly or coconut oil. When the oil is very hot, add a handful of henna leaves and allow it to splutter till it becomes red. Remove the burnt leaves from the oil and once again add to the same oil, a fresh handful of leaves, which will again splutter and turn red. Remove the burnt leaves and repeat the process for two or three handfuls more. Then allow the oil to cool, and bottle. Massage the head with this oil twice a day for 40 days. (*Note:* The burnt and blackened leaves obtained during the preparation of this oil can be powdered and used as a medicine for the treatment of burns, wounds, etc.)

✤ Fungal infection affecting the web of the toes (athlete's foot)

: Take 1 tbsp finely ground paste of henna leaves along with 1 tsp turmeric powder. Mix in 1 tsp gingelly oil. Use this ointment on the affected toes.

✤ Gonorrhea

: Use a decoction of leaves as a douche.

✤ Haemorrhoids

: Grind 1 tsp cleaned henna leaves with 1 cup water. Strain and allow to stand for 15 minutes. Drink 1/2 cup twice a day.

✤ Headache

: Soak a handful of flowers or 2 tbsp crushed seeds in 3 cups of water for a few hours and wash the face with the infusion frequently.

✤ Heaviness in the head

: Grind together the leaves of henna, tamarind and dhatura (*D. alba* or *D. fastuosa*). Make a thin mixture with water, heat in a large potsherd and apply as a warm plaster along the length of the spine.

✤ Insomnia

: Tie a bunch of flowers in a muslin cloth bag and leave the bag near the pillow while sleeping. (*Note:* This treatment is also reported to bring down excessive heat in the body.)

✤ Insomnia, body-heat, prolonged headache

: Soak a handful of henna flowers in 1 cup coconut oil. Massage the head well before going to bed.

✤ Itch, syphilis

: Soak 3 tsp leaves overnight in water. Remove the leaves and drink the infusion for 20 days.

: Grind 2 tsp leaves along with 6 black peppercorns, 1 garlic clove and $1/4$ tsp turmeric into a fine paste. Mix this paste in 1 cup milk. Add sugar to taste and take this beverage every morning for 1 week.

❧ Jaundice, *pitta*-aggravation
: Soak 2 or 3 tbsp root bark in a pot of water and from it frequently.

: Crush $1 1/2$ tsp cleaned henna leaves and boil in 2 cups water till the volume is reduced to 1 cup. *Dose:* $1/2$ cup twice a day.

❧ Joint pain
: Apply the oil extracted from the seeds.

❧ Leprosy (early stages)
: Take equal quantities of the juices of the tender leaves and flowers. Boil this mixture of juices till the volume is reduced by half. *Dose:* 2 tsp thrice a day.

❧ Leucoderma
: Grind the root bark with milk and apply on the affected areas.

❧ Mouth-ulcer
: Boil 2 tbsp leaves in 1 teacup water. Cool. Gargle 3 to 4 times a day.

❧ Pox
: Grind the leaves and apply the paste on the soles and feet. (*Note:* It is believed that this treatment during the disease will save the eyes and eyesight from undue ravaging.)

❧ Ringworm
: Grind a handful of cleaned leaves along with 1 tsp pure, mild soap powder

(*Note:* No detergent to be substituted) into a very fine paste. Apply this on the affected areas and leave it on for at least half an hour. Take a cold water bath.

✦ Sore throat : Boil 1 tbsp leaves in 1 teacup water. Filter and use the decoction for gargling frequently.

✦ Syphilis : Make a paste of 2 tsp leaves, one garlic pod and 5 black peppercorns and eat for 5 days continuously on an empty stomach. (*Note:* During this treatment, no salt should be included in the diet.)

✦ Weeping eczema : Powder 2 tbsp root bark and mix into it 4 tbsp coconut oil and store. At the time of application, add 1 tsp castor oil and wait for an hour before applying with the help of a bird's feather.

✦ Wounds : Wash the wounds with a decoction, of leaves.

Note: Individual results may vary.

In Science

Bhatnagar, S. S. et al. 1961. Biological activity of Indian Medicinal Plants. Part I. Antibacterial, anti-tubercular and antifungal action. *Indian J. Med. Res.* 49:799–813. (Extract of henna leaves are effective against the following bacterial strains: *M. pyogenes, D. pneumonae, B. subtitlis, E. coli, S. typhi, V. choleriae* and *S. dysenterial.*)

Central Council for Research in Ayurveda and Siddha. 1996.

Pharmacological Investigations of Certain Medicinal Plants and Compound Formulations used in Ayurveda and Siddha. New Delhi. p. 223–225. (Analgesic and anti-inflammatory effects proved in laboratory experements; decoction of bark showed marked protection against liver damage in rats.)

Chopra, R. N. et al. 1956. *Glossary of Indian Medicinal Plants.* New Delhi: Council of Scientific and Industrial Research. 151. (Fights jaundice, spleen enlargement, skin diseases, leprosy, headache and sore throat.)

Gupta, S. et al. 1990. An anti-inflammatory agent from *Lawsonia inermis* (Henna) stem bark. Abstract. *Intl. J. Toxicology Occup. Envtl. Health* 1(1):237. (Controls swelling.)

———. 1993. Valuation of anti-inflammatory activity of some constituents of *Lawsonia inermis. Filoterap.* 64(4):365–366.

Hemadri, K. and S. S. Rao. 1983. Anti-fertility, abortifacient and fertility promoting drugs from Dandakaranya. *Ancient Sci. Life* 3(2): 103–107. (Fresh root paste mixed in rice-wash terminates pregnancy.)

Islam, S. N. et al. 1991. Screening of the leaf extracts of *Lawsonia alba* against clinically resistant isolates of *Shigella* and *Vibrio cholerae. J. Bangladesh Acad. Sci.* 15(1):77–80. (Antibacterial properties documented.)

Jain, J. P. and V. N. Pathak. 1970. Antifungal activity of leaf extracts of certain plants. *Labdev. J. Sci. Technol.* 8B(1):58. (Antifungal activity against *Diplodia natalensis.*)

Mishra, S. S. and S. N. Dixit. 1979. Antifungal activity of leaf extracts of some higher plants. *Acta Bot. Indica.* 7(2): 147–150. (Antifungal action noted.)

Munshi, S. R. et al. 1977. Anti-fertility activity of three indigenous plant preparations. *Planta Med.* 31(1):73–75.

27

Dronapushpi

Leucas aspera

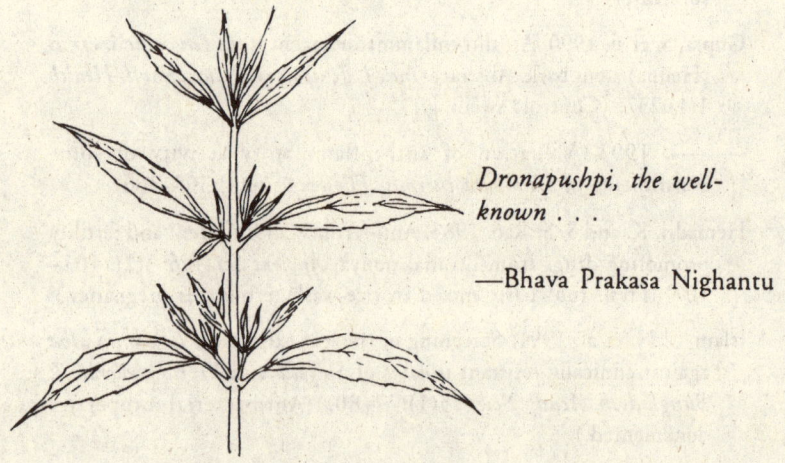

Dronapushpi, the well-known . . .

—Bhava Prakasa Nighantu

The Foot-Shaped Flower

The Tamils call the white flower of dronapushpi *paada-malar*, the flower that is shaped like a foot.

Dronapushpi, like many other medicinal plants, is yet another 'weed' that grows in the wilderness and in wastelands. It is also found in the South East Asian countries and in Bangladesh and Mauritius.

The whole plant is a well-known remedy for fevers, worm infestation, skin diseases and poisonous bites.

Some inhabitants of the South Indian tropical forests believe that the leaf juice of dronapushpi can counteract the poison caused by snakebites. While the flower juice is squeezed into the nostrils of the victim, the leaf is quickly made into a fine paste and the victim is made to eat it. The same paste is applied to the exact spot of the bite as well. In some parts of India, the victim is administered a mixture of half-a-cup each of leaf juice and sesame oil. This treatment induces severe vomiting and diarrhoea, which is believed to flush out the poison accumulated in the system. The traditional treatment includes a condition: the victim of the snakebite is to keep his eyes wide open for as many as 20 hours continuously.

Profile

Botanical Name	:	*Leucas aspera.*	
English Name	:	Thumbe.	
Indian Names	:	Hindi	: *Goma, Motapati, Bara Halkusa*
		Kannada	: *Thumbe, Tummikura*
		Malayalam	: *Tumpa*
		Sanskrit	: *Dronapushpi*
		Tamil	: *Thumbai*
		Telugu	: *Tummachettu*
		Ayurvedic	: *Dronapushpi.*
Family	:	Lamiaceae.	
Appearance	:	Erect herb, 1 to 2 feet tall, with simple, opposite leaves. Flowers, small, white, in axils. Corolla, 2-lipped; upper lip short and hairy and the lower lip twice as long.	
Distribution	:	Found in the Indian plains upto 1000 metres in wastelands. Also found in	

		Bangladesh, Mauritius and in several South East Asian countries.
Medicinal Parts	:	Leaf, flower.
Dose	:	1 to 2 tsp fresh juice twice a day.
Ayurvedic Preparations	:	*Kachoradi Oil, Lasunaghritam, Pathaadigulika,* etc.
Other species	:	*Leucas cephalotes* Spreng.

In Tradition

AILMENTS	PRESCRIPTION
❧ Ague, excessive thirst, eye diseases	: Boil 2 tbsp flowers in 1 cup water till it is reduced to half a cup. Add 1 tsp honey and drink thrice daily.
	: Pluck a whole plant along with its root system. Clean thoroughly in running water. Slice it into small bits and boil in 2 cups of water till reduced to 1 cup. Filter and drink.
❧ Ague, malaria	: Heat a mud pot and toss in a handful of flowers. Add 1 cup water and boil till the volume is reduced to half a cup. Add 2 tsp honey and drink thrice daily.
❧ Amenorrhoea, delay in menstruation	: Grind equal quantities of dronapushpi leaves and uthamani leaves into a very fine paste. Take 1 tsp along with 1 cup milk twice daily. (*Note:* Avoid chillies and tamarind.)

❧ Anaemia, jaundice : Grind equal quantities of the leaves of dronapushpi, keezhanelli and karisilanganni into a very fine paste. Take 1 tbsp with buttermilk in the morning hours.

❧ Asthma : Extract the juice from the fresh leaves and take 2 or 3 tsp. (*Note:* This treatment may induce nausea and sometimes cause vomiting.)

❧ Blockage of nose due to severe cold, catarrh, cephalagia : Squeeze the juice from the leaf into the nostrils.

: Squeeze two drops of flower juice into the nostrils.

❧ Blockage of nose, headache, phlegm : Boil 2 tbsp flowers in $1/4$ cup gingelly oil. When bearably hot, apply on the head.

❧ Diarrhoea and stomach upset in children : Mix in 2 tbsp water, 1 tsp honey and 2 drops each of *Leucas* leaf juice and uthamani leaf juice. Twice daily.

: Mix in 4 drops leaf juice along with 2 drops uthamani leaf juice, 2 pinches black pepper powder and 1 tsp honey. Once or twice a day.

❧ Excessive thirst, fatigue in limbs, headache, heaviness of head, leucorrhoea, phlegm : Cook a handful of leaves along with with greens and a little tamarind. Eat with chapattis or cooked rice.

❦ Eye ailments : Soak 2 tbsp flowers in a cup containing breast milk for half an hour. Use as eye drops. Thrice daily. (*Note:* Apply this milk with a piece of muslin on the forehead and cheeks also.)

❦ Itch, psoriasis, scabies, skin eruptions : Grind the leaves into a fine paste and apply on the affected areas.

❦ Menorrhagia : Grind a handful of leaves into a very fine paste. Squeeze a lime into it and add 1 tbsp gingelly oil, and eat the mixture in the morning on an empty stomach. Continue for 7 days.

❦ Scorpion sting : Mix 4 drops of leaf juice in 1 tsp honey and take. In addition, apply the leaf juice on the puncture caused by the sting.

Note: Individual results may vary.

A Word of Caution

The plant heats up the body. Excessive use is therefore to be avoided.

The plant juice induces vomiting.

In Science

Chandra, K. 1985. Traditional medicine of Baharaich and Gonda districts of U.P. *Sachitra Ayurveda* 37(8):483. (The leaf-paste cures scabies.)

Chopra, R. N. et al. 1956. *Glossary of Indian Medicinal Plants.* New Delhi: CSIR. 153. (*Leucas* is a remedy for cough and cold; it is also a diaphoretic and an insecticide.)

Dhawan, B. N. et al. 1980. Screening of Indian plants for biological activity. Part IX. *Indian J. Exptl. Biol.* 18(6):594. (*L. cephalotes* showed antispasmodic action.)

Kurup, P. N. V. et al. 1979. *Handbook of Medicinal Plants.* New Delhi. P. 64.

Purohit, V. P. et al. 1985. Ethnobotanical studies of some medicinal plants used in skin diseases from Raath (Pann) Garhwal Himalaya. *J. Sci. Res. Pl. Med.* 6(1–4):39. (The leaf-paste is used in the treatment of scabies and skin eruptions.)

Sharma, M. L. et al. 1978. Pharmacological screening of Indian medicinal plants. *Indian J. Exptl. Biol.* 16:228. (The alcoholic extracts of the aerial shoot of the plant exhibited anti-coagulant action.)

Singh, N. et al. 1978. An experimental evaluation of protective effects of some indigenous drugs on carbon tetrachloride-induced hepatotoxicity in mice and rats. *Quart. J. Crude Drug Res.* 16:8. (In this experiment, the plant failed to show any liver-protecting action.)

28

Nagakesara
Mesua ferrea

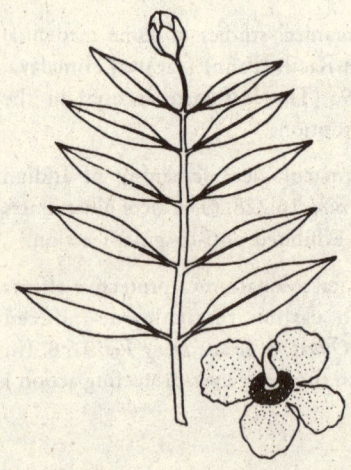

Nagakesara eliminates fevers . . .

—Bhavaprakasam
Karpooradivarga

Ornamental Plant of Many Parts

Nagakesara is an ornamental tree, whose flowers and flower buds are used in folk cosmetics. The aromatic stamens in the flowers are used to stuff pillows and cushions in Malaysia. The dried flowers, along with other aromatics, are used in the preparation of perfumed ointments.

The tree is often cultivated around Buddhist viharas in Sri Lanka. It is considered sacred to Maitreya, the Future Buddha. While its fruits are edible, the seed oil is used in soap-making, lubricating and illuminating. The wood is commonly used in the manufacture of railway sleepers, poles and posts.

In the Unani system, nagakesara is considered a tonic for the heart, and an expeller of wind. It is also used in the Ayurveda and Siddha systems. It is antispasmodic, diuretic and an emmenagogue. In Indonesian medicine, the flowers are used to cure mental illness.

The young fruits contain an oleo-resin from which an essential oil is obtained. It is very fragrant and pale yellow in colour.

The seeds contain a fixed oil which is useful in the treatment of various cutaneous afflictions.

Profile

Botanical Names : *Mesua ferrea* L.
Mesua roxburghii
Mesua coromandalina
Mesua nagassarium (Burm.f.) Kosterm.

English Names : Ceylon Ironwood Tree, Cobra's Saffron, Ironwood.

Indian Names : Andamans : *Gangane*
Assamese : *Dieng-Ngai, Nahor*
Bengali : *Nagesar*
Gujarati : *Nagchampa*
Hindi : *Nagchampa, Nagkesar*
Kannada : *Nagasampige, Nagakesara*
Konkani
& Marathi : *Nagchampe*
Malayalam : *Churuli, Eliponku,*
Nagachampakam,
Nagappoovu, Nanku, Veila,
Veluthapala
Sanskrit : *Champeryah, Nagakesara,*
Nagapushpa
Tamil : *Naangu,*
Nagachambagam,

		Sirunagappoo,
		Velutha champagam,
	Telugu	: *Gajapushpam, Nagkesare, Kesaramu*
	Unani	: *Nagkesar.*
Other Names	Arabic	: *Narae-kaiser.*
	Burmese	: *Gungen, Kengen.*
	French	: *Mesua Naghas.*
Family	:	Guttiferae (Clusiaceae).
Appearance	:	A medium-sized tree with smooth, ash-coloured bark. Leaves, oblong, red when young. They lose their colour very quickly. Flowers, white, aromatic with 4 cup-like sepals. Stamens, many, golden yellow in colour, united to form a fleshy ring. Fruits surrounded by enlarged sepals. Seeds 1–4, angular, brown in colour, smooth. The wood is very hard (and hence the name Ironwood).
Distribution	:	Common in Assam, the Eastern Himalayas, the Eastern and Western Ghats upto about 1500m. Also found in the Andaman islands. Sometimes also a garden plant.
Medicinal Parts	:	Bark, flower buds, flowers, fruits, leaves, oil, root, seeds.
Ayurvedic Preparations	:	*Ashwagandharishta, Chyavanaprasam, Dasamoolarishta, Drakshasava, Lavanabhaskara Churna, Nagakesaradi Churanam, Nagakesara Yoga, Suparipaka.*
Unani Preparations	:	*Hab Pachlauna, Halwa-i-Supari Pak, Jawarish Shehryaran.*

In Tradition

AILMENT   PRESCRIPTION

❧ Bleeding piles : Grind the dried flowers into a very fine powder. Dose: 1/4 tsp with 1 cup warm water.

❧ Bleeding piles, burning sensation in the feet : Grind the dried flowers into a very fine powder. Mix with some ghee and apply externally as an ointment.

❧ Bronchitis, gastritis : Mash 1/4 tsp each bark and root and boil in 1 teacup water. Add 1 tsp honey. Sip.

❧ Cold : Warm the leaves over a flame and apply on head, chest, neck, etc.

❧ Scabies, sores, wounds : Crush 2 cups seeds and express the oil. Apply the oil on the affected areas.

Note: Individual results may vary.

A Word of Caution

The flowers of *Ochrocarpus longifolius* found in the west coast of India are also sometimes referred to as Nagakesara.

In Science

Bhide, M. B. et al. 1977. Studies on anti-asthmatic activity of *Mesua ferrea. Bull. Haff. Instt.* 5:27. (Affirmative results reported.)

Central Council for Research in Ayurveda and Siddha. 1996.

Pharmacological Investigations of Certain Medicinal Plants and Compound Formulations used in Ayurveda and Siddha. New Delhi. (The flowers fight diabetes.)

Chopra, R. N. et al. 1956. *Glossary of Indian Medicinal Plants.* New Delhi: CSIR 166. (A number of pharmacological activities and uses: Astringent, stomachic, cough with expectoration, bleeding piles, burning sensation in the feet, dysentery, snakebite, scorpion sting, etc.)

Dhar, M. L. et al. 1973. Screening of Indian plants for biological activity, Part IV. *Indian J. Exptl. Biol.* 11(1) 43–54. (Ethanolic extracts of the whole plant excluding the root exhibits antibacterial activity against *S. aureus, S. typhi, B. subtilis* and *E.coli.*)

Jain, S. R. and H. R. Jain. 1973. Effect of some common essential oils on pathogenic fungi. *Planta Med.* 24:127. (Seed oil exhibits antifungal activity.)

Kakrani, H. K. 1984. Antimicrobial and anthelmintic activity of essential oil of *mesua ferrea* Linn. *Indian Drugs* 21(6):261–262. (Stamen oil exhibits antifungal activity against *C. tropicalis.*)

Kar, A. and S. R. Jain. 1971. Antibacterial activity of some Indian indigenous aromatic plants. *Flavour Industry* 2:111. (Seed oil effective against *Pseudomonas* sp.)

Seshadri, C. et al. 1981. Anti-fertility activity of a compound ayurvedic preparation. *J. Sci. Res. Pl. Med.* 2(1&2):1–3. (Flowers exhibit anti-implantation activity in female rats.)

Shome, U. et al. 1982. Pharmacognostic studies on the flower of *Mesua ferrea* L. *Proc. Indian Acad. Sci.* 91B(3):211–226.

29

Drumstick

Moringa oleifera

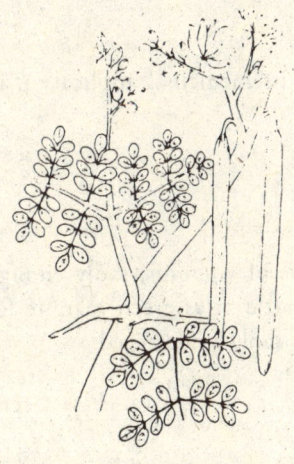

Because of the shape of its fruits, the tree has come to be called 'drumstick'.

The Fruits

The fruits of the drumstick tree are a gourmet's delight in South Indian cuisine and they impart a special flavour to sambar. Highly nutritious, they carry appreciable amounts of proteins, minerals, calcium, iron, phosphorous and Vitamin C. They are also rich in facilitators such as folic acid which help in the absorption of iron, and B-carotene, in the synthesis of Vitamin A.

The Flowers

The creamy-white flowers of the drumstick smell of honey and wood. Folk medicine recognizes the flowers as a powerful aphrodisiac, and they find their way into several jams and concoctions. The flowers are also used in the treatment of several skin-ailments.

The Seeds

The seeds yield an oil which finds its medicinal application in acute rheumatism and gout.

The Leaves

The leaves, a veritable treasure trove of vitamins, sadly enough today end up either as fodder for cattle or as green manure for the soil leaving their rich potential sadly under-used.

The Roots

Drumstick roots also find their use in folk medicines: they are prescribed in the treatment of intermittent fevers, heart ailments, etc.

Profile

Botanical Names	: *Moringa oleifera* Lam. *Moringa pterydosperma* Lam. and Gaertn.
English Names	: Drumstick Tree, Horse-Radish Tree.
Indian Names	: Bengali & Hindi : *Sahinjna, Sahunjana,*

		Sainjan, Sajna,
		Soanjana, Sohanjana,
		Suhunjana
Gujarati	:	*Suragavo*
Malayalam	:	*Saktha, Shakta, Sigru*
Marathi	:	*Shevga*
Punjabi	:	*Soanjana*
Sanskrit	:	*Shobhanjana*
Tamil	:	*Murungai*
Telugu	:	*Munga, Sajana.*

Family	:	Moringaceae.
Appearance	:	A handsome tree with rough and corky bark. Leaves, fern-like, divided and sub-divided. Flowers, white and honey-scented. Fruits, elongated, 3-angular resembling drumsticks. Seeds with wings that facilitate flight to far-flung places.
Distribution	:	Common throughout India.
Medicinal Parts	:	Gum, flowers, leaves, roots, seed oil.

In Tradition

AILMENT	PRESCRIPTION
✤ Anaemia, chest-congestion, senility, sexual debility	: Fry 1/2 tsp black pepper powder in 1 tbsp ghee. Add 2 cups fresh drumstick leaves and stir-fry for 3 minutes. Eat with chapattis or steamed rice for 40 days.
✤ Baldness	: Grind the bark into a very fine paste and apply daily on the patches.

- Blackheads, pimples : Express the juice from fresh leaves and apply on the affected areas frequently.

- Blood-impurities : Add 2 tbsp leaf juice to 1 teacup warm milk. Stir well and drink.

- Blood in urine, gravel in urine : Grind together a handful of roots, bark and 1 tsp black peppercorns into a very fine paste and apply on the abdomen. (*Note:* External application only.)

- Body heat, excessive menstruation, tuberculosis, watery sperm, : Fry 1 cup very tender fruits in 2 tbsp ghee and eat for a month.

- Cataract, prevention of : Grind 100 corns each of drumstick seeds and black pepper into a very fine paste. Smear it on a brass plate and leave under the sun. When the plate is heated, there will be an oily exudate from the paste. Filter through a clean cloth and instil a drop in the eyes. (*Caution:* Take all precautions to prevent avoid infection.)

- Cough, sore throat : Mix a pinch of slaked lime and $1/2$ tsp honey in 1 tsp leaf juice. Apply externally on the throat.

- Diarrhoea : Extract 2 tbsp juice from the leaves and sip with 1 tsp honey. Drink 1 glass tender coconut water.

- Earache : Heat 1 tbsp gingelly oil. Add $1/4$ tsp

gum and allow to come to the boil
and mix with the oil. Cool. When
bearably hot, use as ear drops.

❧ Fatigue : Boil 2 tbsp flowers in 1 cup milk.
Strain and drink.

❧ Fevers : Grind 1 tsp each of the following: black
pepper, dried ginger, *moringa* leaves,
sandalwood paste and vibhitaki. Boil
in 2 cups of water till the volume is
reduced to 1 cup. Drink 1/2 cup of
this decoction along with 1 tsp honey
twice daily.

❧ Headache : Extract the juice from the leaves and
mix with ground black pepper into a
smooth paste. Apply on the forehead.

❧ High blood : Mix 1/2 cup leaf juice with 1/2 cup
pressure, swelling carrot juice and drink.
due to malfunc-
tioning of kidneys,
urine retention

❧ Indigestion, : Extract 2 tbsp juice from the flowers
urine retention and mix with 1 cup buttermilk and
drink.

❧ Pain in joints, : Fry a handful of leaves in 2 tbsp
hips knees, etc. hot castor oil in a skillet. Tie up in a
due to *vata-* muslin cloth and foment the area.
aggravation Repeat.

❧ Swellings : Massage with the oil obtained from the
seeds.

✤ Partial paralysis : Make a soup of 1 cup tender fruits. Add honey and drink for a month.

✤ Pimples : Extract the leaf juice. Mix in an equal amount of lime juice and apply frequently.

✤ Premature ejaculation : Pluck the tender fruits from the tree and cut them into very thin slices. Fry a cupful of these slices in 2 tbsp ghee. Eat with rice or chapattis twice daily for a few days continuously.

✤ Psoriasis, scabies, wounds : Mix equal quantities of leaf juice and gingelly oil and boil thoroughly till the moisture has totally evaporated. Cool and bottle. Apply this oil on the affected parts.

✤ Sexual debility, watery sperm : Boil 2 tbsp seeds in 1 cup milk and drink at bedtime every day for 40 days.

: Boil a handful of drumstick flowers in 2 cups milk and drink at bedtime for a few days continuously.

✤ Semen deficiency : Fry 1 cup leaves in 2 tbsp ghee and eat every day for a few days.

: Steam a handful each of the flowers of coconut, *moringa* and *thudhuvalai* in a pressure cooker. Take along with 2 tbsp each ghee and honey every day for a few days.

❧ Stomach ache : Grind a handful each of the bone-setter (*Cissus quadrangularis*) plant, drumstick flowers and 1 copra (dried coconut) and extract the juice. Drink.

❧ Swelling caused by : Apply the seed-oil after warming it gout, rheumatism slightly on the affected areas.

❧ Urine retention : Grind together 1 tbsp each of the bark in cholera of the drumstick tree, the bark of madar (*Calotropis gigantea*) and black pepper into a very fine paste and apply on the abdomen.

Note: Individual results may vary.

Drumstick Leaf Chutney

Wash a handful of drumstick leaves in running water. Grind them along with 1 onion, $1/2$ inch piece ginger and 1 tsp tamarind pulp into a very fine paste along with salt and green chillies to taste. Eat with cooked rice or chapattis. Remember, the leaves of drumstick contain more B-carotene than any fruit—and that too at a fraction of the cost!

Potato-Drumstick Curry

Roast thinly-diced onion in a little ghee and fry small, whole potatoes along with it. Add curry powder to taste; allow it to cook if necessary with a little water. Add salt to taste. When the potatoes are tender, add a fistful of chopped drumstick leaves and lower the flame. Stir well and eat with cooked rice or chapattis.

In Science

Bhattacharya, S. B. et al. 1982. Chemical investigations on the gum exudate from Sajna *(Moringa oleifera)*. *Carbohydrate Res.* 102:253.

Chatterjee, G. S. and S. R. Mitra. 1951. A note on physiological and chemical findings of the active principle *(Spirochin)* of *Moringa pterygosperma. Sci. & Cult.* 17:43.

Das, B. R. et al. 1957. Antibiotic principle from *Moringa pterygosperma* VII. Antibacterial activity and chemical structure of compounds related to pterygospermin. *Indian J. Med. Res.* 45:191–196.

Eilert, U. et al. 1981. *Planta Med.* 42:55. (About the presence of an active microbial agent in the roots and seeds.)

Ingle, T. R. and B. V. Bhide. 1962. Carbohydrates X. Hydrolysis products of the gum from drumstick plants. *J. Indian Chem. Soc.* 39:623–627.

Joshi, G. V. and I. M. Majumdar. 1959. *J. Univ. Bombay.* 28(46):11. (Aminoacids, amides, organic acids found.)

Kurup, P. A. and P. L. Rao. 1950. Antibiotic principles from *Moringa pterygosperma. Curr. Sci.* 19:43.

Mohan Das, J. 1965. Free aminoacids and carotenes in the leaves of *Moringa oleifera. Curr. Sci.* 34(12):374–375.

Patel, K. C. et al. 1958. Physico-chemical properties of the seed fat of the Moringaceae. *Indian J. Appl. Chem.* 21:85–86. (Seed oil, the traditional medicine.)

Rao, P. L. N. and P. A. Kurup. 1953. Pterygospermin, the antibiotic principle of *Moringa pterygosperma. Indian J. Pharm.* 15(12):315.

Saluja, M. P. et al. 1978. Studies in Medicinal Plants. Part VI. Chemical constituents of *Moringa oleifera* Lamk. (Hybrid variety) and isolation of 4-hydroxymellein. *Indian J. Chem.* 16B:1044–1045.

Sengupta, K. P. et al. 1956. Bacteriological and physiological studies of a vibriocidal drug derived from an indigenous source. *Antiseptic* 53:287–292.

Sreeramulu, N. et al. 1983. *Food Chem.* 1983. 10:205. (Pods and leaves contain Vitamin A, nicotinic acid, ascorbic acid, essential aminoacids; leaves contain Vitamin B; root bark contains an antibiotic principle—pterygospermin.)

30

Sweet Basil

Ocimum basilicum

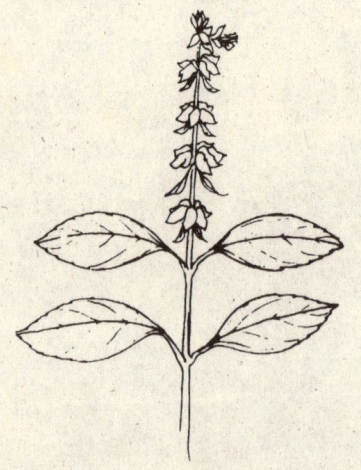

> *Barbari eliminates toxins . . .*
> *and vitiated conditions of*
> *kapha and vata.*
>
> —Bhava Prakasam

The Santhals and Sweet Basil

The Santhals are an ancient tribal community in the northern parts of India, particularly in Bihar and Bengal. Rev. P.O. Bodding, a Norwegian who came to live with the Santhals in the twenties, has published his research work between 1925 and 1940, expatiating on the greatness of their folk-medicine.

Bodding notes in his work the unique method adopted by the Santhals to cope with the searing heat of their homeland: they shake their arms and legs vigorously and rub the soles of their feet with a fine powder of burnt clay. Then they grind sweet basil leaves into a very fine paste and tie it up in a knot in a corner of the dhoti so that the patient is never far from smell of the herb.

Sweet Basil Oil

Sweet basil consists of several varieties. Of them, Curly Leaved Basil is believed to yield a very high-grade oil. In Chalakkudi, Kerala, sweet basil oil is often distilled from the leaves at the time of flowering, when the oil content is reported to be at its peak. The oil possesses insecticidal and insect repellant properties—effective against houseflies and mosquitoes. Its antibacterial properties are well-recognized.

Apart from the leaves, oil is also extracted from the flowers, and this is deemed to be of better quality and value.

The Seeds

The seeds of sweet basil are bitter, cooling, odourless and stimulant. Water extracts of the seeds have in laboratory experiments shown considerable activity against mycobacteria and gram positive bacteria. They are traditionally used in the treatment of dysentery and chronic diarrhoea. They are found useful in vitiated conditions of *vata* and *pitta*. They are also used in the treatment of a host of problems: burning sensations, diarrhoea, dysentery, general debility, haemorrhages, haemorrhoids, sores, wounds, watery sperm, etc. They are also believed to be aphrodisiac.

Sturdy Antibacterial

The leaf and flower extracts of sweet basil have been experimentally found to inhibit the growth of harmful bacteria such as *Micrococcus* spp. While the alcoholic extract of the seeds is also reported to inhibit *Micrococcus* sp, the water extract fights gram positive bacteria and mycobacteria.

Natural Air Freshener

Sweet basil belongs to the family of basils (Labiatae) which includes tulsi as well. The two most distinguishable characteristics of this family are the lip-like corolla and the heavy smell of the leaves.

The characteristic odour of the leaves is due to the numerous dot-like oil glands brimming with volatile oils. The aroma purifies the surroundings, making the basils the most sought after natural air fresheners that are easily grown in the garden. This is perhaps the reason behind the belief that basil ushers happiness into the family that grows it.

Profile

Botanical Name	:	*Ocimum basilicum* L.
English Names	:	Common Basil
		St. Josephwort, Sweet Basil.
Indian Names	:	Gujarati : *Damaro, Nasabo, Sabza*
		Hindi : *Babuitulsi Babul, Baburi Bantulsi, Gulal Tulsi, Barbari, Kali Tulsi*
		Kannada : *Kamakasturi, Ramakasturi, Sajjagida, Tulasi*
		Kashmiri : *Niazbo*
		Malayalam : *Pachcha, Ramatulasi, Tiruneetnu*
		Marathi : *Marva, Subja*
		Oriya : *Dhalatulsi, Kapur Kanti*

Punjabi	:	*Babri, Furrunj, Niyazbo*
Sanskrit	:	*Barbari, Munjaraki,*
		Surasa, Varvara
Tamil	:	*Karpuratulasi,*
		Pachchaitulasi,
		Thirneetru Pachai,
		Vibhudhi-Pachai.
Telugu	:	*Bhutulasi, Rudrajada,*
		Vebhudipatri,
		Vepudupachcha.

Family	:	Labiatae.
Appearance	:	An aromatic herb with green or purplish branches. Leaves, simple, egg-like, shiny. Flowers, 2-lipped, white or pale purple. Fruits, ellipsoid, black in colour.
Distribution	:	Cultivated throughout India.
Medicinal Parts	:	Leaves, the whole plant.
Preparation	:	Infusion (2 tsp of the dried herb in 1 cup water. *Dosage:* 1 cup. *Note:* Add honey, if taken for cough or sore throat).

In Tradition

AILMENT	PRESCRIPTION
❤ Acne vulgaris, pimples	: Expel the leaf juice and apply on the affected areas.
❤ Bad breath	: Gargle with an infusion of the plant.
❤ Body-heat	: Grind the leaves into a paste and tie it up in a handkerchief. Inhale frequently.

215

: Extract 4 tbsp juice from the leaves and mix it into 1 cup milk. Drink every morning for 7 days.

🌿 Boil on the eyelids : Rub a conch shell with the leaf juice of basil and pass gently over the stye.

🌿 Constipation, piles : Crush 1/2 tsp seeds and take with a glass of warm water.

🌿 Earache : Instil 1 or 2 drops of the slightly warmed leaf juice in the ears.

🌿 Earache, infection in the nose : Expel the juice from 2 tsp leaves and instil a few drops into the ears/nose.

🌿 Nasal congestion : Instil 1 or 2 drops of the leaf juice in the nostrils.

🌿 Nasal congestion, phlegm : Finely powder the dried leaf. Use as snuff.

🌿 Sores : Crush the seeds and mix with 1 tsp coconut oil. Apply locally.

🌿 Throat-irritation : Crush the 1 tbsp leaves and extract juice. Mix into 1 cup warm water. Gargle well. (*Caution:* The juice has a slight narcotic effect.)

Note: Individual results may vary.

A Word of Caution

The plant has a slight narcotic effect.

In Science

Bhagat, S. D. et al. 1971. Cultivation of Basil (*Ocimum basilicum* L.) at Jorhat, Assam and the chemical composition of its oil. *Flavour Ind.* 2(8):481–489.

Central Council for Research in Ayurveda and Siddha. 1996. *Pharmacological Investigation of Certain Medicinal Plants and Compound Formulations used in Ayurveda and Siddha.* New Delhi. 464–467. (Anti-implantation activity of the leaf extract noted.)

Chavan, S. R. and S. T. Nigam. 1982. Mosquito larvicidal activity of *Ocimum basilicum* Linn. *Indian J. Med. Res.* 75:220.

Hartwell, J. 1969. Plants used against cancer—a survey. *Lloydia* 32(3):247–296.

Herrera, C. L. et al. 1984. Philippine plants as possible sources of anti-fertility agents. *Philipp. J. Sci.* 113(1-2):91–129. (Anti-fertility properties noted.)

Jain, M. L. and S. R. Jain. 1972. Therapeutic utility of *Ocimum basilicum* var. *album*. *Planta Med.* 22:66 (Anthelmintic activity reported.)

———. 1973. Investigations on the essential oils of *Ocimum basilicum*. *Planta Med.* 24:286. (Anthelmintic action observed.)

Kaul, V. K. and S. S. Nigam. 1977. Antibacterial and antifungal studies of some essential oils. *J. Res. Indian Med. Yoga and Homoeo.* 12(3):132–135. (Fights fungi, especially:*Candida albicans, Candida utilis* and *Aspergillus niger*.)

Khurana, M. L. and M. B. Vangikar. 1950. *Ocimum basilicum* Part II. Antibacterial properties. *Indian J. Pharm.* 12(5):134. (Fights *S. aureus* and *B. typhosa*.)

Kurup, P. A. 1956. Study on Plant Antibiotics: Screening of Some Indian Medicinal Plants. *J. Sci. Industr. Res.* 15C(6):153–154. (Fresh flower extracts exhibit activity against both gram positive (*S. Aureus*) and gram negative (*E.coli*) bacteria.)

Lahariya, A. K. and J. T. Rao. 1979. *In vitro* anti-microbial studies of the essential oils of *Cyperus scariosus* and *Ocimum basilicum*. *Indian*

Drugs 16:150. (Attacks *Proteus vulgaris, Pseudomonas aeruginosa, K. pneumoniae, S. aureus, E. coli, X. campsestris, S.typhae* and *S. paratyphae*. However, the oil did not have any effect on the following bacteria: *B. mycoides, P. mangifera indicae, S. albus* and *V. cholerae*.)

Mukherjee, T. et al. 1984. Herbal drugs of urinary stones (Lit. appraisal.) *Indian Drugs* 21(6):244. (Leaf extract dissolves renal calculi.)

Narayanan, K. et al. 1975. Successful treatment of demodectic mange with a combination of *Erythrina indica, Ocimum basilicum* and *Leucas aspera. Indian Vet. J.* 52:494. (The compound preparation of leaves of two plants, *Ocimum basilicum* and *Leucas aspera* and the seeds of *Erythrina indica* proved an effective cure for parasitic infection by demodectic mange in dogs.)

Naqvi, B.S. et al. 1985. Screening of Pakistani plants for antibacterial activity. *Pakistan J. Sci. Industr. Res.* 28(4):269–275. (Antibacterial activity observed.)

Prakash, A. O. et al. 1978. Effect of oral administration of forty-two indigenous plant extracts on early and late pregnancy of albino rats. *Probe* 17(4):315–323.

Sawhney, S. S. 1977. Antimicrobial efficacy of some essential oils *in vitro. Indian Drugs* 15(2):30–32.

Sharma, S. K. and B. L. Wattal. 1979. Efficacy of some mucilaginous seeds as biological control agents against mosquito larvae. *J. Entomol. Res.* 3(2):172. (Marked larvicidal effects against *Culex* and *Aedes* mosquitoes.)

Singh, R. S. et al. 1986. Dynamics of prime constituent in oil of *Ocimum basilicum* L. *Pafai. J.* 8(2):16–17.

Upadhyay, D. N. and D. N. Bordoloi. 1976. Studies on blight disease of *Ocimum basilicum* Linn. Caused by *Cerespore ocimicoles* Petrole and Oiferi. *Herba Hung.* 15:31–36.

31

Keezhanelli

Phyllanthus amarus

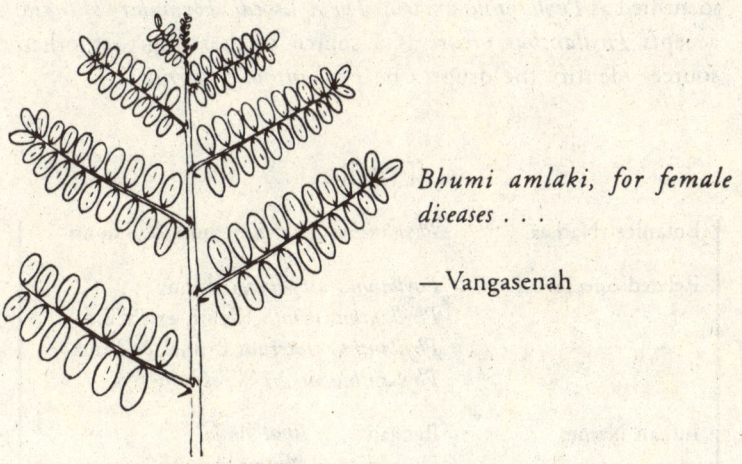

Bhumi amlaki, for female diseases . . .

—Vangasenah

Everyman's Panacea for All Ills

Keezhanelli is a common weed, growing wild in the fields, on the banks of canals and also in wastelands. The leaves of this plant are unusually rich in potassium (0.83% fresh basis) which is considered to be responsible for its powerful diuretic properties. Alcoholic extracts of the leaves and roots show antibacterial activity against *E. Coli* and *M. pyogenes* var. *aureus*. In traditional systems of medicine, the whole plant constitutes the drug. The drug is well-known for its use in the treatment of jaundice. In addition, it is prescribed for colic, diabetes, diarrhoea, dropsy, dysentery, eye ailments, fevers, *pitta*-aggravation, scabies, skin diseases, ulcers, urinary diseases, venereal diseases, etc.

Tamalaki, a commonly available drug in the southern parts of India, is a mixture of two species of Phyllanthus, *P. amarus* and *P. debilis*.

The botanical identity of the plant source with the drug mentioned in ancient texts appears to be unsettled. The drug keezhanelli or tamalaki has, however long been botanically identified as *Phyllanthus amarus. The Ayurvedic Formulary of India* accepts *Phyllanthus niruri* as a source of the drug. Yet other sources identify the drug to be *Phyllanthus fraternus*.

Profile

Botanical Names	:	*Phyllanthus amarus* Schum & Thonn.
Related Species	:	*Phyllanhus airy-shawii* Linn. *Phyllanthus debilis* Kleinn ex. Willd *Phyllanthus fraternus* Brunal & Roux. *Phyllanthus niruri* Webster.

Indian Names	:	Bengali	: *Bhui Amla*
		Gujarati	: *Bhonya Anmali*
		Hindi	: *Jaramla, Jungli Amla, Jungli Amli*
		Kannada	: *Kiranelligida, Kirunelli, Nelanelli*
		Malayalam	: *Keezhaarnelli, Kilaanelli, Kilukanelli, Kirganelli, Kirutaanelli*
		Marathi	: *Bhui Avala*
		Oriya	: *Bhui Aola*
		Sanskrit	: *Bahupatra, Bhumyaamlaki, Tamalaki*
		Tamil	: *Keezhanelli, Keezhakkanelli*
		Telugu	: *Nelausirika.*

Family	:	Euphorbiaceae.
Appearance	:	Annual herb with closely arranged leaves. Flowers, minute, yellowish-green in clusters. Seeds, 6, black, triangular, with longitudinal ribs.
Distribution	:	A native of America and now a circumtropical weed. It is common in cultivated fields, gardens and wastelands.
Medicinal Parts	:	The whole plant, leaves, roots.
Ayurvedic Preparations	:	*Chyavanapraasa Leham, Chemparutyaadi Tailam, Amritapraasa Ghritam, Madhuyastyaadi Tailam.*

In Tradition

AILMENT		PRESCRIPTION
❧ Amenorrhoea, leucorrhhoea, menorrhagia	:	Dry equal quantities of the root of keezhanelli, the bark of ashoka and anjir trees and powder. *Dose:* 1/2 tsp along with 1 cup hot water twice daily for 40 days.
❧ Blood in the urine, burning sensation during urination, dryness of skin	:	Grind 1 tbsp keezhanelli along with 2 tbsp durva grass into a very fine paste. Mix with 1 cup buttermilk and take every morning.
❧ Body-heat, fevers	:	Boil 1/2 cup of keezhanelli (containing both roots and leaves) along with 4 black peppercorns in 2 cups water. Filter and drink thrice a day.

❧ Constipation : Coarsely powder the following: 2 tsp root of keezhanelli, 6 dried rose petals, 1 tsp tail pepper, 4 tbsp cardamom seeds, 2 tsp cumin and 5 tbsp raisins. Add 8 cups water and boil till the solution is reduced to one-fourth of its original volume. *Dose:* $1/2$ to 1 cup along with 1 tsp powder of palm sugar.

❧ Dysentery : Grind 1 tsp each of the leaves of keezhanelli and the tender leaf-buds of pomegranate into a fine paste and drink with buttermilk.

: Boil 1 tbsp leaf-buds of keezhanelli along with $1/2$ tsp fenugreek seeds in 1 cup water. Filter and drink the decoction.

❧ Eyesight deficiencies : Boil 1 cup each of the juices of keezhanelli and *Ponnaanganni* in 2 cups gingelly oil till all traces of moisture disappear. Cool and bottle. Massage the head with this oil for 20 minutes and wash off every day. Continue for a month or two.

❧ Gonorrhoea : Take 1 tbsp each of the whole plants of tulsi and keezhanelli and mix with 1 cup yoghurt and take twice a day for a few days.

❧ Headache, mucus discharge through nostrils : Boil 1 tbsp of the juices of each of the following; leaves of keezhanelli, Indian acalypha, and *Kurutaka* in 3 tbsp gingelly oil till all traces of water are eliminated. Store the powdery residue in a bottle and use as snuff.

✤ Itch : Pluck a handful of leaves and grind them with 1 tsp salt and apply on the affected areas.

: Dry the leaves. Grind them into a fine powder. Use this powder as a soap substitute for washing and bathing.

✤ Jaundice : Grind equal quantities of the leaves of keezhanelli, *Ponnaanganni (Illicebrum sessile)* and dronapushpi. *Dose:* 2 tsp paste along with milk twice daily for a few days. (*Note:* During this treatment, sour and hot foods like chillies, tamarind, etc. are to be avoided.)

: Wash a whole keezhanelli plant thoroughly in running water to remove soil particles, etc. Add 2 cardamoms and 2 tail peppercorns. Now add a glass of water and boil thoroughly till the original volume is reduced to one-fourth. Dose: $1/4$ cup twice daily.

: Crush 5 whole keezhanelli plants (after washing them thoroughly in running water) along with a handful each of Vishnukranti *(Evolvulus alsinoides)*, Bhringaraja *(Eclipta)*, 2 tsp each cardamom and cumin and $1/2$ cup raisins. Add 2 litres of water and boil the mixture till the original volume is reduced to one-fourth. *Dose:* $1/2$ to 1 cup, twice daily.

❧ Jaundice : Take a whole cleaned keezhanelli plant, 2 tail peppercorns and 2 cardamoms. Crush to make a paste. *Dose:* 1 tsp with buttermilk or milk twice daily.

: Crush a whole plant after cleaning well. Mix into a glass of milk. Filter and drink.

❧ Oedema, ulcer : Boil 1 cup rice in 3 cups water and skim off the frothy starch from the grains. Add a fistful each of the roots and leaves of the keezhanelli and 1 tbsp salt to the starch and boil. Use this pulpy broth as a poultice.

❧ Skin diseases : Grind a fistful of the leaves along with 1 tbsp salt into a fine paste. Use as a poultice.

Note: Individual results may vary.

In Science

Bhatnagar, S. S. et al. 1961. Biological activity of Indian medicinal plants. Part I. Antibacterial, antitubercular and antifungal action. *Indian J. Med. Res.* 49:799. (Antifungal activity against *Helminthosporium sativum.*)

Bhowmick, B. N. 1982, Antifungal activity of leaf extracts of medicinal plants on *Alternaria alternata* (Fr) Keissler. *Indian Bot. Rep.* 1:164. (Active.)

Central Council for Research in Ayurveda and Siddha. 1990. *Phytochemical Investigations of Certain Medicinal Plants Used in Ayurveda.* New Delhi. 203–204. (Chemical evaluation of plant properties.)

Dalziel, J. M. 1948. *The Useful Plants of West Tropical Africa*. London: Crown Agents for the Colonies. 157. (African ethno-botany.)

Dhar, M. L. et al. 1968. Screening of Indian plants for biological activity. Part I. *Indian J. Exp. Biol.* 6:232. (Anti-cancer and antispasmodic properties.)

Dixit, S. P and M. P. Achar. 1983. *Bhumyamalaki (Phyllanthus niruri* L.) and jaundice in children. *J. Natl. Integ. Med. Assocn.* 25(8): 269–272. (Fights infective hepatitis in children.)

Nadkarni, K. M. 1954. *Indian Materia Medica*. Bombay: Popular Book Depot. 948. (Medicinal use.)

Ramakrishnan, P. N. et al. 1982. Oral hypoglycaemic effect of *Phyllanthus niruri* Linn. leaves. *Indian J. Pharm. Sci.* 44:10. (More effective than tolbutamide.)

Sivarajan, V. V. and I. Balachandran. 1994. *Ayurvedic Drugs and their Plant Sources*. New Delhi: Oxford & IBH. p.466–467.

Syamsunder, K. V. et al. 1985. Antihepatotoxic principles of *Phyllanthus niruri* herb. *J. Ethnopharmacol.* 14:41. (Fights toxicity in the liver.)

Thiagarajan, S. P. et al. 1982. *In vitro* inactivation of HBsAg by *Eclipta alba* Hassk. and *Phyllanthus niruri* Linn. *Indian J. Med. Res.* (Suppl.) 76:124.

Vimala Devi, M. et al. 1986. Effect of *Phyllanthus niruri* on the diuretic activity *punarnava* tablets. *J. Res. Edn. Indian Med.* 5(1):11–13.

32

Katurohini

Picrorhiza kurroa

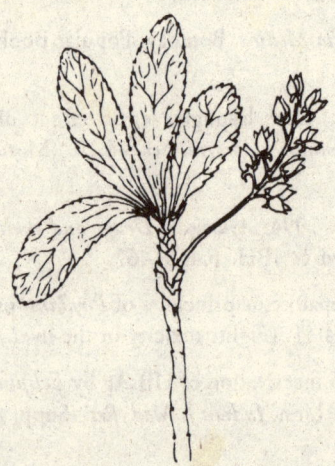

Katurohini drives away fevers . . .

—Bhavaprakasa Nighantu

The Yellow Gentian's Medicinal Uses

Katurohini or the yellow gentian, native of the highlands, is found in the alpine Himalayan mountains at about 3000 to 4000m altitude. It is extensively used in the Ayurveda, Siddha and Unani systems of medicine. The drug comprises the dried rhizomes.

In the Siddha and Ayurveda systems, it is used in the treatment of fevers, asthma, stomach ailments and leprosy.

In the Unani system, katurohini finds its use in the treatment of kidney stones, epilepsy, dog-bite, paralysis, etc. It is also used as an emetic and is a favoured component in eye-lotions for improving eyesight.

External application of a fine powder of katurohini is found to be effective in the treatment of skin diseases. The powder also possesses antibiotic properties.

It is used in the treatment of general weakness, fatigue, loss of appetite, indigestion, liver diseases, jaundice, hysteria, etc.

Its antibiotic activity has been ratified in laboratory conditions.

The Chemistry of the Drug

The drug contains a bitter glycoside (Kutkin). It also contains a non-bitter product (Kurrin), vanillic acid, a sterol (Kutkisterol), an alcohol (Kutkiol) and an odorous principle, sesquiterpene. It is a recognized substitute for the European Gentian, *Gentiana lutea* L.

Profile

| Botanical Names | : *Picrorhiza kurroa* Royle ex Benth. |
| | *Picrorhiza scrophulariiflora* Pennell. |

| English Name | : Yellow Gentian. |

Indian Names	:	Bengali	: *Kataki, Kuru*
		Gujarati	: *Kadu*
		Hindi	: *Katki, Katuka, Kutki, Kuru*
		Kannada	: *Katukarohini*
		Kashmiri	: *Karu*
		Malayalam	: *Kadugrubani, Katurohini*
		Marathi	: *Kutaki*
		Punjabi	: *Kali Kutki*
		Sanskrit	: *Katuka, Katurohini, Katvi*
		Tamil &	
		Telugu	: *Kadugu-Rohini*.

Family	:	Scrophulariaceae.
Appearance	:	Small, hairy perennial herb with woody rootstock. Flowers, pale, white to bluish purple. Leaves, spatula-shaped.
Distribution	:	Grows in the Alpine Himalayas from Kashmir to Sikkim at an altitude of 3000 to 4000m.
Medicinal Part	:	Rootstock.
Ayurvedic Preparations	:	*Katukadaya Lauha, Tikatadi Kvatha, Tikatadi Ghee.*
Unani Preparation	:	*Maajun Jograj Guggal.*

In Tradition

AILMENT	PRESCRIPTION
❧ Ascites	: Boil 1 tsp finely-powdered rootstock in 1 glass water till it is reduced to $1/4$ glass. Take this decoction once every day for a few days. (*Note:* The treatment can induce 4 to 5 motions a day.)
❧ Body weakness	: Take 3 to 5 pinches of the powder of the dried rootstock along with $1/2$ tsp sugar twice a day.
❧ Constipation	: Mix 3 to 5 pinches of the powder of the rootstock along with $1/2$ tsp of any of the following: salt, pepper, asafoetida or *Triphala.*
❧ Constipation, dyspepsia	: Mix 3 to 5 pinches of finely powdered rootstock along with $1/2$ tsp sugar in

228

$1/2$ cup warm water. Take on an empty stomach during the morning hours.

❖ Eye infections : Dust $1/2$ a pinch of powdered rootstock into the affected eyes.

❖ Feverishness : Take 5 to 7 pinches of the powder along with 1 tsp sugar 3 times a day.

❖ Jaundice : Add 4 tsp each of the following: katurohini, calamus, raisins and the bark of a very old neem tree to 4 cups water. Boil thoroughly till reduced to 1 cup. *Dosage:* 2 tbsp twice daily.

: Mix $1/4$ tsp each of the powders of katurohini and turpeth and take along with some sugar and hot water.

❖ Jaundice, convulsions, fever, stomach ache : Powder equal quantities of the following: katurohini, black pepper, rind of bitter orange (dried), sandalwood and cumin. Put 1 tsp of this mixture into a tea pot containing 2 cups boiling water and cover. Filter after a while. *Dosage:* 2 to 4 tbsp twice daily.

❖ Liver problems : Take $1/4$ tsp powdered root along with 1 tsp honey three times a day.

❖ Skin diseases : Mix 1 tsp powder with sufficient juice extracted from tulsi leaves to form an ointment-like consistency. Apply on the affected areas frequently.

Note: Individual results may vary.

A Word of Caution

Excess intake of katurohini can cause dysentery.

As the drug is very bitter, it is usually advised that it be mixed with other ingredients such as black pepper, asafoetida, salt, sugar, etc.

In Science

Ahuja, G. L. 1990. *Hridroga* (diseases of heart) and other treatments in Ayurveda with my practical experience of 5 years. *J. Nat. Int. Med. Assoc.* 32(3):9–11.

Chaturvedi, G. N. and R. P. Singh. 1964. A clinical study on the causes of jaundice and its treatment with an indigenous drug, *Picrorhiza kurroa* Royle and its preparation. *J. Med. Sci.* 5:9. (Effective in the treatment of jaundice.)

Dwivedi, Y. et al. 1990. Hepato-protective activity of Picroliv against carbon-tetrachloride-induced liver damage in rats. *Ind. J. Med. Res.* 92B:195–200.

Khan, A. B. and A. Shahid. 1985. Effect of *Picrorhiza kurroa* Benth. on experimental liver damage induced in rats. Thanjavur: Tamil University. *Symposium on Traditional Medicine.* p 61.

Pandey, V. N. and G. N. Chaturvedi. 1968. Effect of alcoholic extract of *Katura (Picrorhiza kurroa)* on experimentally induced abnormalities in the liver of rabbits. *J. Res. Indian Med.* 3,2:25–35.

Rajalakshmi, S. et al. 1992. Effect of *Kadugurohini (Picrorhiza kurroa* Royle) in the treatment of viral hepatitis—A double blind study with placebo control. *J. Res. Ayur. Sid.* XIII, 1&2:27–34. (The bile salts and bile pigments went down to nil after 14 days treatment; definitive action of the drug in the process of clearance of viral hepatitis.)

Singh, G. B. et al. 1993. Anti-inflammatory activity of the iridoids, kutkin, picroside-1 and kutkoside from *Picrorhiza kurroa*. *Phytotherap. Res.* 7(6):407. (Anti-fertility activity reported.)

33

Long Pepper

Piper longum

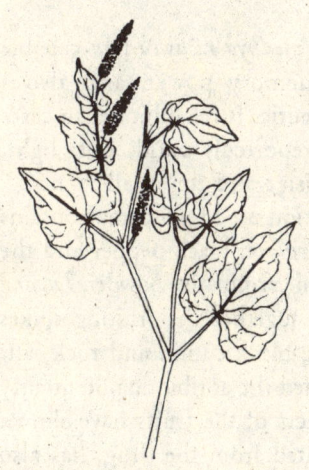

> *With a paste of pippali, several poisons can be destroyed.*
>
> —Matsya Purana
> 218.20. (8th century A.D.)

'The First Medicine'

Long pepper, which consists of the dried fruits of the plant, is referred to as *Aadi Marundu* (the original or first medicine) in Tamil. The fruits which are used generally as a spice and also in pickles in Indian cuisine have a pungent pepper-like taste and produce salivation and numbness of the mouth. The plant is called long pepper as its spikes are longer and therefore distinguishable from black pepper. *Pippalimoolam* or the roots are also used in Ayurvedic medicine. In some hilly parts of Visakhapatnam district in Andhra Pradesh, the plant is grown for its roots, used in the preparation of fermented rice beer.

The plant's name in Sanskrit, *magadhi,* refers to its original habitat : Magadha, present-day North Bihar. Here, it grows near water sources and streams as a creeper.

In traditional medicine, it is used to cure headache, cough, throat-problems, respiratory diseases, bronchitis, ENT-ailments, eye diseases, gas problems, indigestion, colic, piles, physical weakness, dyspnoea, ascites, leprosy, diabetes, piles, cardiac and spleen disorders, worm infestation, etc.

In Ayurveda, it is an important *medhya rasayan* i.e., capable of improving the intellect and memory power, and also a prophylactic and post-illness therapeutic. It rehabilitates in cases of vitiated *vata* and *kapha.* It is reportedly acrid, hot, light, digestive, and an appetiser, aphrodisiac and tonic, all in one.

Piplarishta, an Ayurvedic preparation used for asthma contains long pepper, bark of *Symplocos paniculata,* black pepper and the stem of *Cissampelos pareira.* A common carminative powder, *Lavana Bhaskara* is prepared by powdering together the fruiting spikes and roots of long pepper, coriander, black cumin and rock salt.

Recent experiments have confirmed the antibiotic potentiality of the leaves and fruits. Ether extracts of the fruits have shown larvicidal properties. Piperine, isolated from the drug, has also exhibited anti-tubercular activity. Regular intake of one pod of long pepper along with 1 cup milk every day is considered to be a potent anabolic by some herbalists.

In the Andaman Islands, the leaves are chewed like betel leaves.

Profile

Botanical Name	:	*Piper longum* Linn.
English Names	:	Long Pepper, Indian Long Pepper
Indian Names	:	Assamese : *Piplu*

Bengali	: *Jatya, Pipul, Piplamur (root)*
Gujarati	: *Pipli*
Hindi	: *Pipal, Pipli, Piplamool (root)*
Kannada	: *Hippali, Tippali*
Malayalam	: *Tippali, Magadhi, Pippali*
Marathi	: *Pimpli*
Sanskrit	: *Pippali, Magadhi*
Tamil	: *Pipili, Tippili*
Telugu	: *Modi, Pipalu, Pipili*
Unani	: *Filfil-a-Suyah, Filfil-Sarah, Filfil-a-Suya Pipalkalan*
Jalpaiguri	: *Shwappa.*

Family	: Piperaceae.
Appearance	: Trailing or creeping aromatic plant. Leaves, dark green and shining above but pale on lower surface. Stipules, conspicuous but soon drop off. Fruit, small, ovoid, sunk in fleshy spike. Spike, 2 to 4 cm long, oblong, blackish green, shining.
Distribution	: Grows in the warmer regions of India, particularly in Assam, Uttar Pradesh, West Bengal and in the southern parts of the country.
Medicinal Parts	: Dried fruits (*Pippali*), roots (*Pippali-moolam*).

Dose: 5 to 10 pinches of root powder with honey, ghee or sugar. $1/4$ to $1/2$ tsp root decoction with milk, sugar, ghee or buttermilk. $1/4$ to $1/2$ tsp dry fruit powder along with 1 tbsp honey.

Ayurvedic Preparations	: *Abhayarishtam, Draksharishtam, Chyavanaprasam, Piplarishtam, Pippalyasavam.*
Unani Preparations	: *Itrifal Fauladi, Ma'jun Khadar, Angaruya-i-Kabir.*

In Tradition

AILMENT	PRESCRIPTION
❦ Asthma, bronchitis	: Take equal quantities of the powder of long pepper, dried ginger and black pepper thrice daily.
❦ Cough, fainting, gas problems	: Boil 1/2 tsp powdered long pepper in one glass cow's milk and drink.
❦ Cough, fatigue, sexual debility	: Roast separately: long pepper—1 teacup; black pepper and dried ginger— 1/2 teacup each; cumin, black cumin, lesser galangal, ajwain, cinnamon leaves, cloves (*Syzigium aromaticum*), cardamon, *Chitraka (Plumbago zeylanica)* and *triphala*—all 1/4 teacup each; and cinnamon bark— 1/8 teacup. Powder. Add the required quantity of honey. Take half-a-teaspoon of this mixture for 40 days.
❦ Cough, hiccups, sinus congestion, sore throat	: Add to 1 teacup boiling water 1/2 tsp each ground long pepper, cloves and rock salt, and let the mixture steep for 10 minutes. Filter, and drink while still warm.
❦ Diarrhoea	: Take the powder of 1/2 tsp long pepper along with warm water.
❦ Fatigue, sexual debility	: Mix equal quantities of the powders of long pepper and chebulic myrobalan. Add some honey. Take 1 tsp twice a day for 1 or 2 months.

♦ Hiccups,   : Mix 1/2 tsp each finely ground pippali,
  vomiting   juice of matulunga (*Citrus medica*) and
                      sugar with 1 tsp honey and swallow.

♦ Influenza   : Mix 1/2 tsp powder of long pepper with
  (preliminary stages) 2 tsp honey and 1/2 tsp juice of ginger.
                      Take thrice a day.

♦ Throat infection : Roast the following: Tail pepper—
                      6 tbsp; liquorice, long pepper, *Suganda
                      vacha* (*Alpinia officinarum*) and rind of
                      Haritaki (*Terminalia chebula*)—3 tbsp
                      each; cardamom—1 tsp. Powder and
                      store in a bottle. Boil 1/4 tsp in 1/2
                      cup water. Add milk and honey and
                      drink.

♦ Tinea versicolor : Take 1/2 tsp long pepper powder along
                      with honey for 40 days.

In Science

Annamalai, A. R. and R. Manavalan. 1990. Effects of Trikatu and its individual components and piperine on gastro-intestinal tract. *Indian Drugs* 27:595–604.

Anshuman, P. S. et al. 1984. Effect of *vardhaman pippali* (*Piper longum*) on patients with respiratory disorders. *Sachitra Ayurved* 37(1):47–49.

Atal. C. K. et al. 1966. Occurence of sesamin in *Piper longum* Linn. *Indian J. Chem.* 4:252.

————— et al. 1975. Chemistry of Indian *Piper* species. *Lloydia* 38:256. (Piperidine isolated.)

Bhargava, A. K. and S. C. Chauhan. 1968. Antibacterial activity of essential oils. *Indian J. Pharm.* 30:150. (Antibacterial properties recorded.)

HOME REMEDIES

Bisht, B. S. 1963. Pharmacognosy of 'Piplamul'—the root and stem of *Piper longum* Linn. *Planta Med.* 11:410–416. (Medicinal importance.)

Chopra, R. N. et al. 1956. *Glossary of Indian Medicinal Plants.* New Delhi: Council of Scientific and Industrial Research. p. 194. (Long pepper as an antidote to scorpion sting and snakebite.)

Das, P. C. et al. 1983. Use of *Piper nigrum* and *Piper longum* as anti-malarial drugs. Bombay: *Asian Conference of Traditional Asian Medicine.* (Anti-malarial role of piperine.)

Dehanukar, S. A. et al. 1984. Efficacy of *Piper longum* in childhood asthma. *Indian Drugs* 21(9):384–388.

Dhar, K. L. and C. K. Atal. 1967. Occurence of N-isobutyldeca trans-2 trans-4-dienamide in *Piper longum* Linn. and *Piper peepuloides* Royle. *Indian J. Chem.* 5:588–589.

Khan, R. S. et al. 1999. Effect of Trikatu, an ayurvedic preparation, on the pharmacokinetic profile of carbamazepine in rabbits. *Indian J. Physiol. Pharmacol.* 43(1):133–136.

Koul, I. B. and A. Kapil. 1993. Evaluation of the liver-protective potential of piperine, an active principle of black and long peppers. *Planta Medica* 59(5):413–417.

Kulshresta, V. K. et al. 1969. A study of central stimulant effect of *Piper longum. Indian J. Pharm.* I:8 (Respiratory stimulation in dogs.)

———. 1971. The analysis of central stimulant activity of *Piper longum. J. Res. Indian Med.* 6:17. (Respiratory depression overcome.)

Kurup, P. N. V. et al. 1979. *Handbook of Medicinal Plants.* New Delhi. (Antitubercular properties studied.)

Lee, E. B. et al. 1984. Pharmacological study on piperine. *Arch. Pharm. Res.* 7(2):127–132.

Manavalan, R. and J. Singh. 1979. Chemical and some pharmacological studies on leaves of *Piper longum* L. *Indian J. Pharm. Sci.* 41:190–191. (Leaves as medicine.)

Shoj, N. et al. 1986. Dehydropiperonaline, an amide-possessing coronary vasco-dilating activity isolated from *Piper longum* L. *Jour. Pharm.*

Sci. 75(12):1188–1189. (Dried fruits display coronary vasodilating activity.)

Singh, N. et al. 1970. *Piper longum* induced rat hind paw oedema, a new method of detecting anti-inflammatory activity. *J. Res. Indian Med.* 5(1):130. (Anti-inflammatory.)

Singh, N. et al. 1973. Studies on analeptic activity of some *Piper longum* alkaloids. *J. Es. Ind. Med.* 8:1.

Shin, K. H. et al. 1984. Pharmacology of piperine. Seoul: *Proceedings of the Fifth Asian Symposium on Medicinal and Aromatic Plants and Spices.* August 20–24. p. 219. (Activities reported: CNS depressant, analgesic, anti-pyretic and anti-inflammatory.)

34

Castor

Ricinus communis

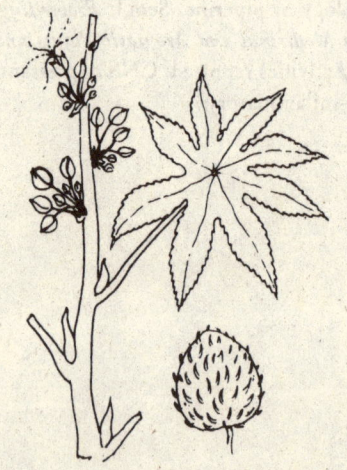

Oil of castor, an effective purgative . . .

—Priya Nighantu

From the Dark Continent

Castor originated in Africa, and it was quite popular with the early Egyptians. The plant is widely grown in Morocco to anchor sand dunes.

Excavations from several pyramids dating from 4000 B.C. have shown castor seeds, indicating that it could have been an important item of commerce in ancient Egypt and enjoyed pride of place in royal households.

Castor in Ancient Indian Texts

Sushruta Atharvaveda, an Indian text written in 2000 B.C. mentions two varieties of castor: white and red-seeded.

The Leaves

The castor plant is raised in Assam to feed the *Eri* silkworm. The leaves are occasionally fed to cattle in order to increase the milk yield. The powdered leaves are useful in repelling mosquitoes, white flies and aphids.

The Seeds

The seeds are the source of castor oil, which is used in transparent soaps, typewriter ink, aromatics, paints and varnishes. The seed cake is used as a fertilizer. While the wood pulp of the plant is used in paper making, the stems make straw-boards and wrappings.

The Oil

Medicinally, castor oil is a strong purgative. It is used in the preparation of several medicated oils (*Siddha Taila*). It is cathartic, demulcent, analgesic and nervine. Laboratory tests indicate its anti-inflammatory role (Sharma et al. 1969; Dhar et al. 1968). They also stand testimony to its analgesic (Gupta et al. 1982; Tewari and Chaturvedi, 1981) and anti-viral action (Singh and Singh, 1972).

Profile

Botanical Name	:	*Ricinus communis* L.
English Names	:	Bofareira, Castorbean, Castor Oil Plant, Mexico Seed, Palma Christi.
Indian Names	:	

Assamese & Bengali	:	*Bherenda*
Gujarati Hindi & Marathi	:	*Diveli*
	:	*Arandi*
Kannada	:	*Haralu, Manda, Oudla*
Malayalam	:	*Avanakka*
Oriya	:	*Jada*
Sanskrit	:	*Eranda, Panchaangula*
Tamil	:	*Amanakku, Kottaimuthu*
Telugu	:	*Erandamu*
Andhra (Krishna dist.)	:	*Pedda Amadam.*

Family	:	Euphorbiaceae.
Appearance	:	A tree-like shrub, herbaceous, 3 to 10 feet tall. Leaves, palm like. Fruit, spiny capsule. Seeds, glossy.
Distribution	:	Cultivated chiefly in Andhra Pradesh, Maharashtra, Karnataka and Orissa.
Medicinal Parts	:	Leaves, seeds, roots, oil obtained from the seeds.
Varieties	:	White-seeded *bhat-rendi* and pale-seeded *jogia-rendi.*

In Tradition

AILMENT	PRESCRIPTION
✤ Arthritis, boils, rheumatism, swellings	: Cut the leaves into thin shreds. Fry them in hot castor oil. Apply on the affected parts when bearably hot.
✤ Bed sores	: Crush the fresh leaves of Indian acalypha in 2 tbsp castor oil. Apply on the affected parts when bearably hot. Leave on for half an hour at the very least.
✤ Body ache, muscular pain	: Fry a few leaves of *Indravalli (Cassyta filiformis)* in a little castor oil and eat.
✤ Boils	: Crush a castor leaf and fry in a little castor oil. When bearably hot, tie it on with a bandage.
	: Warm a betel leaf over a flame till it becomes soft. Coat it with a layer of warm castor oil and spread over the inflamed parts.
	: Burn the stem of dhatura in burning coal and collect its ash. Add a little castor oil to make a paste. Apply on the affected areas.
✤ Boils, sores, swellings	: Warm the leaves over a flame and bandage.
✤ Boils, swellings	: Fry crushed castor leaves in coconut oil. Pack in a muslin cloth and foment the affected parts.

❧ Boils, to quicken
their ripening

: Warm a betel leaf over a flame till it is soft and pliable. Apply warm castor oil on its surface. Spread over the affected parts and allow it to remain for a few hours. Repeat, if necessary.

❧ Cracks in nipples

: Apply castor oil locally.

❧ Dandruff

: Regular use of castor oil as hair-oil.

❧ Dry skin

: Massage the whole body with castor oil once a week; apply castor oil on the hands and feet at bedtime.

❧ Eye diseases

: Instil 1 or 2 drops of the infusion of the leaves in the eye. (*Caution:* Take all precautions to prevent infection.)

❧ Flatulence in
children

: Warm the leaves coated with oil over a flame and apply over the abdomen.

❧ Guireaworm sores

: Apply pounded leaves to extract the worm.

❧ Headache, boils

: Use a poultice of leaves.

❧ Heaviness
in the stomach and
to eject hardened
lumps of stools

: Take 2 tbsp castor oil in a glassful of milk at bedtime. After a few motions, take 2 tsp fleaseed with 1 teacup curd, three times a day. (*Caution:* This treatment should not be undertaken frequently.)

❧ Hiccups

: Mix 2 parts honey with 1 part castor oil. Take $1/2$ tsp at a time. (*Caution:* Excess intake may cause purgation.)

❧ Orchitis

: Take the mature kernel of coconut (a

half-portion). Grate well, and fry it in a little castor oil with 2 tbsp crushed garlic. Eat once a day for a few days. (*Note:* This can be mixed with steamed rice or eaten with bread or chapattis.)

❧ Pain in eyes, burning sensation in the eyes
: Apply castor oil over the eyelashes before going to sleep.

❧ Pain in the lower abdomen
: Apply warm castor oil on the lower abdomen. Fry some bits of castor leaves in castor oil and apply when bearably hot.

❧ Redness in eyes due to pollution or due to medication
: Mix a little breast-milk in castor oil and apply on the eyes at bedtime.

❧ Rheumatic and gouty swellings
: Fry mashed castor seeds in a little castor oil. Pack in a muslin cloth and apply on the affected areas as a poultice.

❧ Rheumatic joints
: Use a poultice of seeds or leaves.

❧ Stomach ache
: Soak bits of leaves in water for an hour and drink the infusion.

❧ To increase lactation
: Warm the leaves and apply over the breasts as poultice.

: Massage the breasts frequently with warm castor oil.

❧ To increase lactation in nursing mothers
: Fry bits of the leaves in a little castor oil. When bearably hot, tie on the breasts. Leave on for 30 to 40 minutes.

✤ Toothache : Massage the gums with root paste and rinse out with warm water.

✤ Whitlow : Blend castor oil and milk cream (1:1) and apply. Bandage firmly.

Note: Individual results may vary.

A Word of Caution

The entire castor plant, including its seeds, contains an irritant which is toxic to the blood. The seeds are poisonous and even 2 or 3 seeds can be fatal. Although local medical systems prescribe the intake of one seed per day to prevent pregnancy in women, it is advisable not to follow such practices. The oil is however considered free of any toxic substance. Repeated use of castor oil is not advisable as in some people, it has caused secondary constipation i.e. re-occurrence.

Persons suffering from renal disorders should not use castor oil internally.

Castor oil intake, in excess, may cause abortion and hence pregnant women are not advised to consume it.

Use of castor oil as a facilitator in childbirth, although widely practised in villages, has doubtful results.

Castor oil is sometimes adulterated with rosin oil, cotton seed oil, lard, etc.

In Science

Chopra, R. N. et al. 1956. *Glossary of Indian Medicinal Plants.* New Delhi: Council of Scientific and Industrial Research. 214. (Use in scorpion sting.)

Chowdhary, R. R. et al. 980. Review of plants screened for anti-fertility activity. Part III. *Bull. Medico-Ethno-Bot. Res.* 1(4):542–545. (Promising anti-fertility role.)

Dastur, J. F. 1951. *Useful Plants of India and Pakistan.* Bombay: D. B. Taraporevala Sons & Co. Ltd. p. 201.

Dhar, M. L. et al. 1968. Screening of Indian plants for biological activity. *Indian J. Exp. Biol.* 6(4):232–247. (Anti-inflammatory.)

Garg, S. K. 1974. Anti-fertility effects of oil from a few indigenous plants on female albino-rats. *Planta Med.* 26(4):391–393.

Gupta, R. A. et al. 1982. Screening of Ayurvedic drugs for analgesic activity. *J. Sci. Res. Pl. Med.* 3(4):115–117. (Analgesic.)

Huh, I. et al. 1983. Effect of L-adrenergic drugs and other drugs on castor oil induced diarrhoea in rats. *Yakhak Hoeji* 27(4):368.

Kamboj, V. P. and B. N. Dhawan. 1982. Research on plants for fertility regulation in India. *J. Ethno-Pharmacol.* 6(2)191–226. (Anti-fertility use ratified.)

Kirtikar K. R. and B. D. Basu. 1935. *Indian Medicinal Plants.* 4 Vols. Allahabad: Lalit Mohan Basu. III:2273

Mahl, B. S. and V. P. Trivedi. 1972. Vegetable anti-fertility drugs of India. *Quart. J. Crude Drug Res.* 12(3):1922–1923.

Nadkarni, K. M. 1954. *Indian Materia Medica.* Bombay: Popular Book Depot. 3rd edn. 2 Vols. I:1065.

Sakurai, E. et al. 1991. Diarrhoea and biogenic amines: Regional changes and serotonin metabolism following castor-oil induced diarrhoea in rats. *Yakugaku Zasshiv* III (4,5):241–246.

Sharma, V. N. et al. 1969. Anti-inflammatory activity of *Ricinus communis* Linn. (*Eranda*) *J. Res. Indian. Med.* 4:47.

Singh, P. 1956. Pharmacognostic study of root of *Ricinus communis* L. *J. Sci. Industr. Res.* 15:259–262. (Medicinal value of the root.)

Singh, R. and R. Singh. 1972. Screening of some plant extracts for anti-viral properties. *Technology* (Sindri) 9:4:415–416. (Fights many a virus.)

Tewari, P. and C. Chaturvedi. 1981. Methods of Population Control in Ayurvedic Classics. *Ancient Sci. Life* 1(2):72–79.

35

Rose

Rosa centifolia

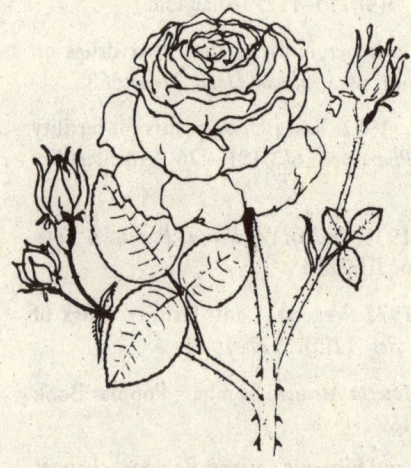

Satapatri, ideal for skin diseases . . .

—Dhanvantari Nighantu

The Versatile Herb

Roses cultivated in gardens for ornamental purposes are complex hybrids derived from numerous wild species. Their numbers run into several thousands. New types are created ceaselessly by rose breeders.

A few species are grown on a commercial scale for the preparation of products like itr, rose oil, rose water, etc. which are widely used in perfumery and medicine.

Paleontologists have found fossils of roses which are thought to be over 30 million years old. Archaeolgists have discovered paintings of roses which once adorned the frescoes of Cretan palaces and Egyptian tombs. The Chinese have been cultivating roses since as early as 2737 B.C. They also developed the tea-rose strains in their gardens with the aroma of freshly brewed tea.

Folk-practitioners of medicine were not far behind. They too found in roses both the food and the medicine ideal for human beings.

The Flower of Love

Rose is valued as the flower of love. The Romans, fascinated by the beauty and sensuousness of these flowers, wore them in wreaths; realizing their nutritive and medicinal value, they added them to their puddings, jellies, honey and sundry other dishes. Even while drinking their wine, as a toast to a friend, they plucked a petal and put it into their goblets. Their rooms and furniture were strewn with roses; they put rose blossoms into their bathtubs to help preserve the skin and after bathing massaged their bodies with rose ointments; they slept in beds of petals.

Along with the Roman empire, the use of the rose also appears to have suffered a downfall. It took several centuries before roses retrieved their lost glory.

The Middle Ages witnessed the convents and monasteries growing roses chiefly for medicinal use. They were used to cure earaches and toothaches.

Rose Hips

Rose hips, which are the remnants after the petals wither away and fall, were used in Great Britain during the Second World War as a supplement to citrus fruits, which were in short supply. They were made into a syrup and given to growing children.

It is indeed amazing that a mere 100gm of rose hips contains as much as 150mg of ascorbic acid (Vitamin C). Compare this with 50mg in fresh orange juice, 20mg in raw tomatoes and a mere 5mg in raw apples.

A virtual gold mine of Vitamin C!

Profile

Botanical Name	:	*Rosa centifolia* Linn.
English Names	:	Cabbage Rose, Hundred-Leaved Rose, Pale Rose, Rose.
Indian Names	:	Bengali : *Golap* Hindi : *Gulab* Kannada : *Gulabi* Malayalam : *Paninirpuvu* Sanskrit : *Satapatri, Saumya Gandha, Vritta Pushpa* Tamil : *Paninirpoo, Roja* Telugu : *Gulabi, Rojappuvu.*
Chinese Name	:	Yeu Ji Hua.
Appearance	:	Prickly shrubs, white to crimson flowers. Stems bear alternate, odd-pinnate leaves. Flowers are usually single and five-petalled in wild species, but are often double in the cultivated varieties.
Distribution	:	Cultivated chiefly in Aligarh, Ghazipur and Kanauj, though widespread throughout India.
Medicinal Parts	:	Flowers, hips.

In Tradition

AILMENT	PRESCRIPTION
❦ Anaemia	: Boil 6 tsp each crushed fennel seeds and red rose petals in $1^1/_2$ cups water, strain and drink twice daily.
❦ Angina pectoris	: Thoroughly mix 1 tsp rose oil with 4 tsp sweet almond oil. Rub on the chest, morning and evening.
❦ Blood impurities, nervousness, weak heart	: To an infusion of 2 tsp flowers in 1 glass water, add 1 tsp honey and drink.
❦ Burning sensation in the eyes	: Instil several drops of pure rose water in the affected eye.
	: Mix 1 tsp each rose water and onion juice. Drench clean cotton in this liquid and place on the closed eyes.
❦ Burns, wounds	: Apply the decoction as above on the affected areas.
❦ Blood diseases, heart problems, nervousness	: Add 1 tsp honey to an infusion of dried rose petals and take every morning for a few days.
❦ Cataract in the early stages	: Mix rose water and lime juice (3:1). Use as eye drops.
❦ Constipation	: Eat gulkand (see the recipe), frequently.
	: Eat 6 tsp gulkand with milk.

- Diarrhoea (esp. for children) : Add a handful of petals in a glassful of water, raise to the boil and allow to stand 15 minutes before serving.

- Diarrhoea, piles stomach upset : Boil a handful of rose petals in a glass of water and take 2 or 3 times a day.

- Dizziness, headache : Take an infusion made of dried rose petals (1 tbsp) and 1 cup boiling water.

- Dysentery : Grind 2 tsps rose leaves with $1/2$ cup water. Strain. Drink twice daily.

- Epiphora : Dissolve a pinch of alum in 2 tsp rose water. A wad of cotton-wool soaked in it can be used as dropper.

- Fever : Wash the patient's forehead with cold water to which rose water and vinegar have been added.

- Haemorrhoids : Pat the anus with rose water to soothe.

- Headache : Use rose petals as a cold compress for the forehead.

  : Mix finely powdered tail pepper and dried ginger (*Sonth*) (1 tsp each) in a little rose water and apply on the affected area.

- Heart problems : Take 2 tsp gulkand (see Rose: Some Derivatives) every day.

- Insomnia : Thoroughly mix rose oil (3 drops), violet oil (3 drops) and sweet almond oil (4 tbsp) and preserve. Apply to the scalp, ears and soles of the feet before

250

sleeping. Apply a small amount to the anus as well.

❧ Intestinal ulcers : Boil 2 tsp flowers in 1 glass water. Take the decoction frequently.

❧ Mouth-ulcer : Wash the mouth frequently with a decoction of rose petals.

: Gargle with a decoction of dried rose petals frequently.

❧ Nausea and vomiting during pregnancy : Take a mixture of gulkand (2 tsp) and pomegranate juice (1 cup).

❧ Sexual debility : Mix equal parts of rose hips, rose buds, tea leaves and jasmine flowers. Steep 2 tbsp of the mixture in 1 cup boiling water for 10 minutes. Sweeten with 1 tsp honey and drink.

❧ Sore throat : Add a few dried petals to honey and chew frequently.

: Take rose-honey. (see Rose: Some Derivatives.)

❧ Tachycardia : Steep in diluted rose water, 1 tsp aniseed, $1/2$ tsp coriander seeds and 10 raisins overnight. Strain and drink the following morning.

❧ Threatened abortion : Gulkand of petals of white rose in 2 to 3 tsp doses every day.

❧ Toothache : Gargle with a decoction of dried rose petals to which 1 tbsp wine is added.

ROSE: Some Important Species

Rosa californica: Californian Rose
Spanish-Americans are very fond of the ripe hips either raw or stewed.

Rosa centifolia: Cabbage Rose
It is the source of commercial rose water. The infusion, powder and tincture are reported to be useful for haemorrhage.

Rosa damascena: Damask Rose
Source of the attar of roses, it is used as a rejuvenating agent and is said to be helpful in regulating the menstrual cycle. It also helps to induce sleep.

Rosa gallica: French Rose
Its infusion is used as vaginal douche or as an eyewash.

Rosa laevigata: Cherokee Rose
In China, it is used to treat problems of frequent or excessive involuntary release of semen.

Rosa roxburghii
In China, its hips are used to cure dyspepsia.

Rosa moschata (Wild Himalayan Hill Rose)
They grow throughout the Himalayas.

ROSE: Some Derivatives

1. *Dried Petals*
Petals to be dried are collected much before the flower unfolds. They are rapidly dried in the shade below 50°C. Dried petals, popularly known as *pankhuri* are used during the hot weather for preparing cold drinks.

2. *Rose Water*
Fresh petals are boiled in water and the vapour is condensed in another vessel to get rose water. For internal use, a dose is 2 tbsp. It rejuvenates the mind and heart and is cooling and refreshing to the eyes. It controls inflammations such as conjunctivitis.

3. *Rose Tincture*
Add 1 glass boiling water to 2 tbsp dried petals. Add 10 drops of oil of vitriol and 4 to 5 tsp white sugar. Strain. Take 3 to 4 tsp twice or thrice a day for haemorrhage or as a stomachic.

4. *Rose Vinegar*
Steep rose petals in distilled vinegar. Don't boil. A cloth soaked in rose vinegar can be used as a compress for headaches.

5. *Rose Honey*
Pound fresh petals in a little boiling water. Filter and boil the liquid with honey. This is a heart and nerve tonic. It is also a blood-purifier, and an ancient remedy for sore throat.

6. *Gulkand*
Layer fresh petals with honey and sugar and allow the mixture to mature for a fortnight. This taken at bedtime in milk as a mild anti-*pitta* laxative, especially for the heat of summer. It also helps relieve excessive menstrual bleeding.

7. *Gul Roghan*
A hair-oil prepared from rose petals by enfleurage with wet sesamum seeds (Rose petals are mixed with wet sesamum seeds so that the fragrance is absorbed by the seed-mass). Limited quantities of this product are prepared in Uttar Pradesh.

8. *Itr (Rose Attar)*
This extract of roses is based on paraffin or sandalwood oil.

253

Rose-Based Moisturizer

You can make your own moisturizer with hardly any trouble, and free of industrial preservatives:

All you need is some rose water and glycerine (1:1 ratio). Mix them thoroughly and bottle. Use in place of commercial moisturizers.

In Science

Gopalaswamiengar, K. S. 1951. *Complete Gardening in India*. Bangalore: The Hosali Press. 309. (Popularity of the Edward rose in India.)

Guenther, E. 1948–1952. *The Essential Oils*. New York: Von Nostrand. 6 Vols. V:25.

Gupta, R. K. 1968. *Flora Nainitalensis*. New Delhi: Navayug Traders.

Kirtikar, K. R. and B. D. Basu. 1935. *Indian Medicinal Plants*. Allahabad: Lalit Mohan Basu. 4 vols. 2nd edn. II: 983. (Rose hips cure wounds, sprains and ulcers.)

Nadkarni, K. M. 1954. *Indian Materia Medica*. Bombay: Popular Book Depot. 2 Vols. I:1073.

Narayanaswami, V. and K. Biswas. 1957. *Survey of Rose-Growing Centres and Rose Industry in India*. New Delhi: CSIR.

Naves, Y. R. and G. Mazuyer. 1947. *Natural Perfume Materials*. New York: Reinhold.

Pal, B. P. 1972. *The Rose in India*. Revised edn. New Delhi: ICAR.

Parry, E. J. 1921–1922. *The Chemistry of Essential Oils and Artificial Perfumes*. London: Scott, Greenwood & Son Ltd. 2 Vols. I:391.

Poucher, W. A. 1959. *Perfumes, Cosmetics and Soaps*. London: Chapman & Hall. 3 Vols. 6th edn. II: 212.

Sairam, T. V. 1997. Rose, The Flower of Love, *Dignity Dialogue* 3(2): 32–39.

Venkataratnam, L. 1960. *Horticulture in Central India.* New Delhi: Ministry of Food & Agriculture 161.

Sharma, M. L. 1986. Extraction of rose oil from flowers. *Indian Rose* A5:162–169.

Sharma, M. L. et al. 1987. Damask Rose. In *Ecodevelopment of Alkaline Land: Banthra—A case-study.* Ed. T. N. Khoshoo. Lucknow: National Botanical Research Institute. 83–86.

Srivastava, H. P. 1986. Perfumery roses on alkaline lands. *Indian Rose* A5:170–176.

Uphof, J. C. Th. 1968. *Dictionary of Economic Plants.* Verlog Von J. Cramer. 2nd edn. 454. (In Iran, flowers are used to treat colic and diarrhoea.)

36

Tamarind

Tamarindus indica

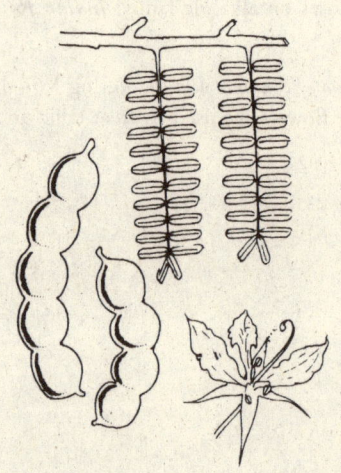

Vrkshamla, one among the ten cardiac tonics . . .

—Charaka

The Date Palm of India?

Arab travellers who came to India called the tamarind tree 'The Date of India' (*Tamar-i-Hind*), although the tree has its roots in Africa.

Villagers in India believe that the tree houses spirits and hence nobody will sleep under its shade; the tree, according to them, will prevent even a blade of grass from growing by it.

A Must on the Sailor's Shopping List

In olden days when continents were connected only by sea-routes, the tamarind invariably found its place foremost on every sailor's shopping list. The reason: its tang prevented sea-sickness and nausea. Today we know that its antimicrobial and antibacterial properties must have also protected them from the deadly tropical germs that abound in the coastal areas. Perhaps this quality of tamarind lies behind the wise Indian's use of tamarind juice in preparing the daily meal for the family.

The Pulp

The fruit pulp is the chief flavouring agent in curries, chutneys and sauces. It is perhaps one of the most acidic naturally occuring substances, the principal acid being tartaric acid.

Apart from its use against germs, the fruit pulp also exhibits several medicinal properties: anthelmintic, carminative, digestive, laxative and refrigerant. It is considered to be a useful liver tonic as well. It is used in rural households as a powerful utensil cleaner, particularly for burnishing brass and silver utensils.

The Leaves

The leaves too fight worms; their juice is used in the treatment of bleeding piles.

The Bark

The bark of the tree possesses astringent and antipyretic properties.

Profile

| Botanical Name | : | *Tamarindus indica* L. |
| English Names | : | Indian Date, Tamarind, Tamarindo. |

Indian Names	:	Bengali	: *Tentul*
		Gujarati	: *Ambli*
		Hindi	: *Amli, Ampli, Imli, Tentul*
		Kannada	: *Chinch, Huli, Amli*
		Malayalam	: *Amlam, Kolpuli, Puli,.* *Pulimaram, Valampuli*
		Marathi	: *Ambli, Chinch*
		Oriya	: *Tentuli*
		Sanskrit	: *Amlika, Chincha, Tintrini*
		Tamil	: *Puli*
		Telugu	: *Amlaki, Amlika, Chinta,* *Chintachettu.*

Family	:	Leguminoseae.
Appearance	:	A tree with small, shiny leaflets. Flowers, creamy yellow to pinkish, in clusters. Pods, thick and oblong. Seeds, brown, compressed, embedded in a fibrous, fleshy, acid pulp.
Distribution	:	Native of tropical Africa, the tree is quite common in India.
Medicinal Parts	:	Bark, flowers, fruits, leaves (tender), seed kernel.

In Tradition

AILMENT	PRESCRIPTION
✤ Biliousness, constipation, dyspepsia, flatulence	: Grind some tender leaves into a fine paste. Add a little salt and eat with cooked rice.
✤ Bleeding piles, dysuria	: Extract the juice from 1 cup leaves and apply on the affected parts.

❧ Blood clot due to injuries, congelation of blood

: After removing the seeds and fibre, mix the pulp (3 tbsp) with 1 tsp salt and 1/2 cup water. Mix thoroughly and heat the mixture in a container. When bearably hot, apply on the affected areas. Wash with water the next day and repeat for 3 days.

❧ Body-heat, indigestion, loss of appetite, tastelessness

: Rasam, either drunk or with plain, steamed rice. (See recipe below)

❧ Burns caused by hot liquids, oil or water

: Sprinkle finely powdered tamarind bark on the open wound and drizzle drops of coconut oil over it.

❧ Cold, cough

: Boil a handful of tamarind flowers in 2 cups water till the volume is reduced to 1 cup. Filter. *Dose:* 1/2 cup twice a day for 2 days.

❧ Constipation

: Steep 1 tbsp tamarind pulp and 1 tsp senna overnight in 1 cup water and strain. Add 1 tbsp gulkand and eat the next morning.

: Boil the fruit pulp (2 tsp in 1 glass water) and drink when lukewarm.

❧ Cough, throat problems

: Boil a handful of leaves in 2 cups water till the volume is reduced to 1 cup. Allow the filtrate to cool. Use for frequent gargling.

❧ Dysentery, slimy stools

: Collect the seeds and crush them. Gather the brownish broken bits and dry fry in a frying pan till they turn reddish in colour. Now grind them into a very fine powder and bottle. *Dose:* A pinch of this powder to be taken with 1 tsp honey thrice daily.

❧ Earache, excessive urination : Boil 1 tsp leaves in 2 tsp gingelly oil. Cool and use the filtrate as ear drops. Grind together equal quantities of the leaves of horse radish along with the kernel of tamarind seeds and the required quantity of water. Warm and apply the paste on the pelvic region.

❧ Eye diseases : Grind a handful of cleaned flowers into a fine paste and apply around the eyes at bedtime.

❧ Fatigue : Collect the most tender leaf buds and cook along with lentils. Temper $1/2$ tsp cumin in 1 tsp ghee and add. Mix well and eat with steamed rice or chapattis once a day for a few weeks.

❧ Fevers : Make an infusion of 1 tsp fruit pulp in 1 cup water and drink.

❧ Fever due to *pitta*, nausea : Mix into 1 tsp tamarind pulp (diluted) 1 tsp palm sugar and $1/4$ tsp powdered black pepper. Dilute further with $1/2$ cup warm water and drink.

❧ Gum inflammations : Mix 1 tsp pulp with $1/2$ tsp salt and press on the affected parts.

❧ Heaviness of head : Grind 2 tbsp each of the leaves of tamarind, henna and dhatura along

260

with 1 tsp salt into a very fine paste. Dilute with $1/2$ teacup water. Boil and when hot and paste-like in consistency apply as a plaster around the head. Tie a cotton napkin tightly around the head and retire.

❧ Indigestion : Boil a handful of flowers in 2 cups water till the volume is reduced to 1 cup. Add 1 tsp palm sugar and drink.

❧ Intestinal worms : Grind a handful of tamarind leaves along with a little salt and 1 green chilly into a very fine paste. Eat this chutney with steamed rice or chapatti.

❧ Itch : Dilute $1/4$ tsp pulp in 1 cup warm water. Mix $1/4$ tsp black salt with it and drink.

❧ Jaundice : Soak overnight 1 tsp tamarind pulp along with 1 tbsp dried alubukhara (plums). Mash in the morning. Add a little black salt and eat.

❧ Joint pains, swellings : Take equal quantities of the flowers and leaves and fry them in castor oil. When bearably hot tie them up in a cloth and foment the affected areas.

❧ Measles : Mix equal quantities of the powders of tamarind seeds and turmeric. *Dose:* 3 to 4 pinches along with hot water thrice a day.

❧ Mouth-ulcer, sore throat : Gargle with an infusion of the leaves.

❧ Nausea in : Chew a tiny piece of tamarind fruit.
   pregnant women

❧ Neuralgia : Boil tamarind leaves with just enough
   water. Transfer to a muslin cloth and
   wring out all traces of moisture. Now,
   foment the affected area as long as the
   leaves retain their warmth.

❧ Painful eyes, : Grind a handful of flowers into a fine
   redness in paste and apply over the eyes before
   eyes going to bed.

❧ Painful swellings : Use a poultice of leaves along with
   neem oil.

❧ *Pitta*-aggravation : Make a paste of a handful of tamarind
   flowers along with some green chillies,
   salt, curry leaves, coriander leaves and
   tamarind. Eat 3 tbsp of this chutney
   with steamed rice or chapattis.

   : Collect the most tender raw from fruits
   and grind them into a paste with some
   salt and green chillies. Eat with steamed
   rice or chapattis for 21 days.

   : Crush a handful of flowers and tender
   leaf-buds along with some pulp, chillies
   and salt and eat with cooked rice or
   chapattis.

❧ Sore throat : Dilute the pulp with warm water and
   gargle.

❧ Scorpion sting : Mix 2 tsp pulp with an equal quantity
   of slaked lime. This produces a hot

mixture which has to be pressed on to the affected area. The patient should also immediately eat the kernel of half a coconut. (*Note:* It is reported that for some people, this treatment does not pay much dividends.)

❖ Swelling due to injuries : Take a lemon-sized ball of tamarind and mash it into thick pulp with some water. Add 1 tbsp salt and boil thoroughly in an iron vessel. Cool and apply on the affected parts.

❖ Swelling in the eyes : Use a poultice of flowers.

❖ Urine retention : Boil a handful of tamarind flowers in 2 cups water till reduced to 1 cup. Filter. Add 1 tsp palm sugar. Drink twice daily.

❖ Watery sperm : Fry tamarind seeds till they turn red. Discard the brown seed-coat and grind the white kernel into a fine powder. Sieve. Bottle. At bedtime, take 1 tsp powder along with 1 tsp candy in 1 cup boiled cow's milk. Repeat this treatment every night for 40 days.

Note: Individual results may vary.

A Word of Caution

Tamarind produces heat in the body. In order to neutralize it, the following spices are added : coriander seeds, coriander leaves, cumin, etc.

Excessive use of tamarind may affect the digestive organs.

Rasam:

Rasam, the hot and tangy soup of southern cuisine can be used as a medicinal formulation, based on the permutation and combination of its constituent spices and condiments.

Step I: Grind the following: 1/2 tsp each cumin seeds, black pepper, coriander seeds, seedless tamarind pulp, curry leaves, garlic paste and ginger paste along with 1 ripe finely cut tomato and a little water. Boil well.

Step II: Fry 1/2 tsp mustard seeds along with a pinch of asafoetida in 1 tsp ghee till it splutters. Add to the boiled mixture.

Eat with plain steamed rice.

In Science

Bremness, L. 1994. *Les Plantes Aromatiques et Medicinales.* (In French) Paris: Bordas. (The flowers reduce blood pressure.)

Burkill, I. H. 1909. *A Working List of the Flowering Plants of Baluchistan.* Calcutta: Superintendent, Government Printing. (Tamarind listed prominently.)

Chopra, R. N. et al. 1958. *Indigenous Drugs of India.* Calcutta: U. N. Dhur & Sons. 2nd edn.

Dastur, J. F. 1951. *Useful Plants of India and Pakistan.* Bombay: Taraporevala Sons.

Howes, F. N. 1949. *Vegetable Gums and Resins.* Waltham: The Chronica Botanica Co.

Kirtikar, K. R. and B. D. Basu. 1935. *Indian Medicinal Plants.* Allahabad: Lalit Mohan Basu. 2nd edn. Vol II.

Kurup, P. N. V. et al. 1979. *Handbook of Medicinal Plants.* New Delhi. 51. (Floral medicine.)

Nadkarni, A. K. 1954. *Indian Materia Medica*. Bombay. 1192. (Flower poultice used in inflammatory affections of the conjunctiva.)

Sambiah, K. and K. Srinivasan. 1991. Effect of cumin, cinnamon, ginger, mustard and tamarind in induced hypercholesterolemic rats. *Nahrung Food* 35(1):47–51.

Sivarajan, V. V. and I. Balachandran. 1994. *Ayurvedic Drugs and their Plant Sources*. New Delhi: Oxford & IBH. 115–116. (In the treatment of constipation, colic, cough, dyspepsia, fever, flatulence, gastro-intestinal and urinary diseases.)

Quisumbing, E. 1951. *Medicinal Plants of Philippines*. Manila: Dept. of Agriculture & Natural Resources.

Whistler, R. L. and J. N. BeMiller. 1959. *Industrial Gums, Polysaccharides and their Devivatives*. New York: Academic Press.

37

Vibhitaki

Terminalia bellirica

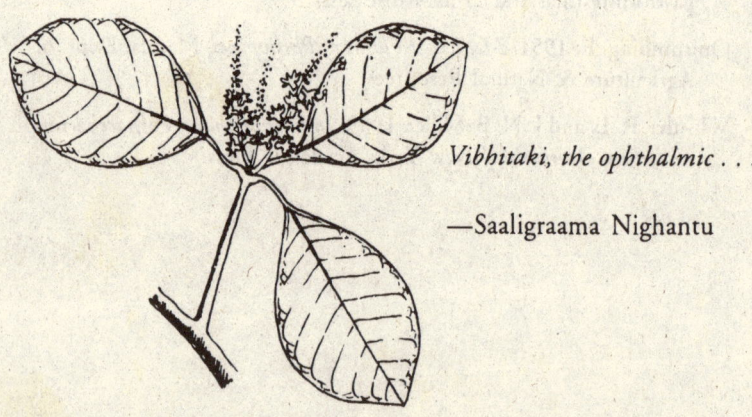

Vibhitaki, the ophthalmic . . .

—Saaligraama Nighantu

One of a Well-Known Trio

The fruits of vibhitaki constitute one of the three ingredients of the famous Ayurvedic preparation, Triphala, which holds pride of place not only in the Indian systems of medicine, but also in the Tibetan system. (The other two ingredients are haritaki (*Terminalia chebula*) and amla (*Emblica officinale*).) In the Unani system, a complete range of products called *Itrifal* contains triphala in addition to various other ingredients, depending upon its final use.

Medicinal Value

The fruits of vibhitaki exhibit hypotensive, purgative and choleretic activities. Its kernel is edible and is considered to have narcotic and aphrodisiac effects.

It is prescribed in a variety of diseases: anaemia, cough, fever, asthma, diarrhoea, dysentery, biliousness, diseases of the eyes, nose and throat, etc. It stimulates hair growth, cures leprosy, and purifies the blood.

Profile

Botanical Names	:	*Terminalia bellirica* (Gaertn.) Roxb. Syn. *Myrobalanus bellirica* Gaertn.
English Names	:	Bastard Myrobalan, Belleric Myrobalan.
Indian Names	:	Assamese : *Bhovian, Hulluch*
		Bengali : *Bhairah*
		Gujarati,
		Hindi,
		Marathi &
		Punjabi : *Bahera*
		Kannada : *Tandrikayi, Santikayi, Bahera, Vibhita, Tari*
		Malayalam : *Taani, Taanikka*
		Marathi : *Beheda*
		Oriya : *Bhara*
		Sanskrit : *Telaphala, Vibhitaki, Beheduka, Aksha, Akshaya*
		Tamil : *Taanikkai, Akkam, Tanri, Vibeedagam*
		Telugu : *Tandra, Tadi, Tandri, Taani Vibhitakamu.*
Family	:	Combretaceae.
Appearance	:	A large avenue tree with ash-grey bark,

with patches of blue. Leaves elliptic, crowded towards the ends of the branches. Flowers, pale greenish-yellow with an offensive odour. Fruit, grey to light violet when fresh, turning light brown later.

Distribution : Grows wild upto 1000m elevation all over India except in the dry, marshy areas.

Medicinal Parts : Bark, fruits, leaves.

In Tradition

AILMENT	PRESCRIPTION
✤ Breathlessness	: Boil 1 tsp dried fruit in 2 teacups water till the volume is reduced to 1 teacup. Add 1 tsp honey and take once a day.
✤ Cough, sore throat	: Mix equal parts of vibhitaki, long pepper, black raisins, dates, black pepper and honey. Grind them into a fine paste. *Dose:* 1tsp along with 1 tsp honey.
✤ Dry cough	: Make a paste of equal quantities of black raisins, dates, black pepper, vibhitaki, long pepper and honey. Take 1 tsp of the mixture. Repeat 3–4 times a day.
✤ Epiphora	: Grind finely equal quantities of the 3 myrobalans (haritaki, vibhitaki and amla). Mix into this powder twice their

weight of honey and an equal weight of ghee. Take 1 tsp of this mixture twice daily.

❧ Intenstinal worms : Roast the fruit and remove the seeds. Powder the rind. Take $1/2$ tsp with warm water, 3 times a day.

: Mix equal quantities of vibhitaki with the seeds of the flame of the forest (*palas*) and powder. Take 1 tsp of this mixture along with 1 cup hot water thrice a day.

❧ Leucoderma, premature greying of hair, skin diseases : Apply the oil extracted from the seeds locally.

❧ Sore throat : Mix equal quantities of belleric myrobalan, rock salt and long pepper. Take $1/2$ tsp of this mixture along with hot water. (Honey can be added as well.)

: Boil $11/2$ inch bark in 1 teacup water. When bearably hot, gargle.

❧ To impart brightness to the eyes : Roast the rind and powder. Take $1/2$ tsp with 1 tsp each honey and white sugar for three months.

❧ Wounds : Put some crushed myrobalans (*Triphala*) in a potful of water. This water can be used to wash wounds as an antiseptic solution.

Note: Individual results may vary.

In Science

Antarkar, D. S. et al. 1980. Double blind clinical trial of *Arogya Vardhini*—an ayurvedic drug in acute viral hepatitis. *Indian J. Med. Res.* 72:588–593. (Clinical confirmation obtained.)

Burkill, I. H. 1935. *A Dictionary of the Economic Products of the Malay Peninsula.* London: The Crown Agent for the Colonies. Vol. II.

Bhatia, K. et al. 1977. Utilization of bark of *Terminalia* species from Uttar Pradesh. *Indian Forester* 103:273. (The bark is medicinal.)

Chopra, R. N. et al. 1956. *Glossary of Indian Medicinal Plants.* New Delhi: CSIR. 241. (Cures headaches.)

Dhar, D. N. and G. N. Quasba. 1984. Screening of some plant extracts for antifungal activity against *Venturia inequalis*. *Sci. and Cult.* 50(6):209. (The oil is purgative.)

Gaind, K. N. et al. 1964. Anthelmintic activity of *Triphala*. *Indian J. Pharm.* 26(4):106–107. (Water extract of the drug triphala can eliminate worms.)

Godbole, S. H. and G. S. Pendse. 1960. Antibacterial property of some plants. *Indian J. Pharm.* 22(2):39. (The cold water extract of belleric myrobalan exhibits activity against *S. aureus, E. coli* and *E. officinalis*.)

Inamdar, M. C. et al. 1962. Purgative activity of *Triphala*. *Indian J. Pharm.* 24(4):87–88.

Iyengar, M. A. and S. Dwivedi. 1990. *Terminalia bellirica* Roxb (*Bahera*)—A Review. *Indian Drugs 26*(12):655–663.

Kirtikar, K. R. and B. D. Basu. 1935. *Indian Medicinal Plants.* Allahabad: Lalit Mohan Basu. Vol. II.

Miglani, B. D. et al. 1967. Purgative action of an oil expressed from *Terminalia bellirica*: Part XIX. Hyderabad: Indian Pharmacological Congress. *Indian J. Pharm.* 29(12):347.

Mukherjee, G. D. 1976. Principle of treatment of dermatological diseases in Ayurvedic system of medicine. Part 2: The clinical trial (Sc-1) on Vitiligo. *J. Res. Indian Med. Yoga and Homoe.* 11(2):66–69. (Patients suffering from vitiligo respond well.)

Palit, G. et al. 1983. 'Experimental evaluation of anti-asthmatic plant drugs from the ancient ayurvedic medicine.' in *Aspects of Allergy and Applied Immunology.* S. K. Jain (ed.). Indian Coll. of Allergy and Applied Immunology. Delhi: V. P. Chest Institute. XVI, 36–41. (Broncho-dilatory effect recorded.)

Row, L. R. and P. S. Murthy. 1970. Chemical examination of *Terminalia bellirica* Roxb. *Indian J. Chem.* 8:1047.

Tariq, M. et al. 1977. Protective effect of fruit extracts of *Emblica officinalis* Gaertn. and *Terminalia bellirica* Roxb. in experimental myocardial necrosis in rats. *Indian J. Exp. Biol.* 15:465. (In combination with extracts of amla, the drug protects against myocardial necrosis.)

Sharma, R. et al. 1987. Management of tropical pulmonary eosinophilia in children with Ayurvedic drugs. *Jour. Res. Edn. Ind. Med.* 6 (1–2):11–17. (In the treatment of tropical pulmonary eosinophilia.)

Trivedi, V. P. et al. 1982. Clinical study of the anti-tussive and antiasthmatic effect of *Vibhitakphal churnac Terminalia bellirica* Roxb.) in the cases of Kasa-swasa. *J. Res. Ayur. Siddha 3* (1 and 2):1–8. (Bronchodilatory, antispasmodic and anti-asthmatic activities noted.)

38

Haritaki

Terminalia chebula

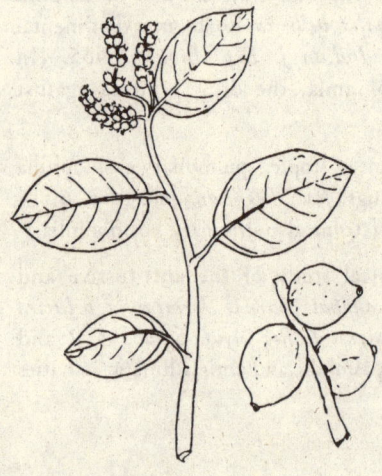

A mother nourishes her baby alone. But the great kadukkai nourishes everybody without distinction. Kadukkai offers protection against diseases as well. Then who could possibly be superior—a mother or kadukkai?

—An ancient Tamil verse

Kaya Kalpa

Haritaki, an indigenous tree of the Indian subcontinent has been in medicinal use from time immemorial.

The fruit constitutes one of the three essential fruits that go into triphala, the well-known Ayurvedic compound. Triphala is a *rasayana* drug, which is dry, hot and potent. It is capable of imparting youthful vitality to the body and greater receptivity to the mind and sense-organs.

The drug induces internal energy and flushes out all nitrogenous and faecal matter from the body. It is thus a great boon to those who suffer from constipation.

It improves the appetite and digestion, tones up the intestinal tissues and strengthens the body. It slows down the ageing process and prolongs life, and enhances the intellect. It is therefore regarded as a *Kaya Kalpa*. It is considered effective in so many ailments that an extensive catalogue is required! Although the ancient texts of Ayurveda recognize 7 varieties of this plant, only 2 survive now: one with normal fruit and the other with smaller fruits (called *Harad Jungli*). Although both varieties possess similar properties, physicians avoid the small fruits.

In Indian medicine 6 kinds of fruits are usually recognized based on their sizes and colour: cumin-like, barley-corn-like, raisin-like, greenish yellow, very nearly mature and fully mature. The second, third and sixth kinds of these are used in medicine and the rest are good only for tanning.

Profile

Botanical Name	:	*Terminalia chebula* Retz.
English Names	:	Black Myrobalan, Chebulic Myrobalan.
Indian Names	:	Bengali : *Haritaki*
		Gujarati : *Hardo*
		Hindi : *Harad, Harara*
		Kannada : *Alalekayi, Harade, Harra, Karakayi*
		Malayalam : *Kadukka*
		Marathi : *Hirda*
		Oriya : *Haridra*
		Sanskrit : *Abhaya, Haritaki, Himaja, Pathya*
		Tamil : *Kadukkai*
		Telugu : *Karakka, Karakayi, Karitaki.*
Family	:	Combretaceae.

273

Appearance	:	Tree with dark brown bark. Leaves, simple, opposite, shiny. Flowers, small, cream-coloured. Fruit, an ellipsoidal drupe, 5-angled, 4 x 2.5 cm.
Distribution	:	Commonly found in North India, chiefly in deciduous forests upto 1000m.
Medicinal Parts	:	Rind of the fruits (raw or dried). (*Note:* The seeds should never be used, as they can prove harmful.)
Ayurvedic Preparations	:	*Triphala, Vishnu Tapa Haran Rasa, Haritaki Hand.*
Unani Preparations	:	*Itriphal, Sharbat Murrakale Musaffi Khun, Ma'ajun Mochras.*

In Tradition

AILMENT	PRESCRIPTION
❦ Acidity, heart-burn	: Grind well 1/2 tsp each of the dried rind of amla and haritaki. Add 1 teacup water and boil the mixture well. Filter and drink along with 1 tsp honey.
❦ Asthma	: Chew a small piece of the dried rind every night.
❦ Bleeding gums, painful gums	: A fine powder of the dried fruit is used as tooth powder.
❦ Body-heat (To remove excess heat from the body)	: Take 1 tsp finely ground powder of haritaki along with 1/2 tsp sugar every morning on an empty stomach for 10 days. After the first 10 days it should be taken twice a day for another 10

days. (*Note:* This treatment will also keep the bowels clean.)

❧ Constipation,

: Take 1 tsp fine powder of the dried rind with a little salt. Chase it down with lukewarm water.

❧ Constipation, loss of appetite

: Take the raw fruits and discard their seeds. Crush the rind into a fine paste. Add salt ($1/5$th of the quantity of crushed fruits). Mix well and store for three months. Take $1/2$ to 1 teaspoonful of this preparation either as such or along with steamed rice.

❧ Dysentery, diarrhoea

: Take $1/2$ tsp of the pulp of the unripe fruit mixed with a little honey and the powder of a $1/2$ inch bit of cinnamon and two cloves twice a day.

❧ Eye disorders, inflammation, redness

: A dilute decoction of the dried fruit as an eyewash.

❧ Greying of hair

: A decoction of the fruit is used as hair-rinse frequently.

❧ Haemorrhoids

: Apply the finely ground powder of the dried rind as such or its decoction on the affected areas.

❧ Headache

: Make a fine paste of the rind and apply on the forehead.

❧ Infection in between the toes, inflammation in the feet

: Finely grind the rind and turmeric(1:1) and apply on the toes before retiring to bed.

275

❧ Inflammation of the eyes
: Make a fine paste of the rind and apply it on the eyelids for 4 or 5 days.

❧ Loss of hair
: Boil thoroughly a paste of 6 fruits in 1 cup coconut oil. Use this hair-oil every day.

❧ Mouth-ulcer
: Make a smooth paste of the powdered fruit with thin buttermilk and use as a mouthwash several times a day.

❧ Mumps
: Grind the fruit with a little water into a thick, smooth paste and apply on affected areas.

❧ Piles
: An unripe fruit is fried in castor oil till it turns golden brown in colour. Powder and store. Take $1/2$ tsp of this powder at bedtime with a little lukewarm water to ensure normal bowel movement. It has a healing effect on piles too.

❧ Vaginitis
: A decoction of dried fruit is used as a vaginal douche. (*Caution:* Pregnant women should not use this.)

❧ Whitlow
: Remove the seeds and roast 6 fruits. Powder. Mix thoroughly with $1/2$ cup diluted tamarind pulp so as to form a paste. Apply the paste on the infected finger at bedtime.

Note: Individual results may vary.

A Word of Caution

Haritaki may not be useful for those who suffer from indigestion, or indulge in dry foods, or undertake fasts or suffer from fatigue, fever, phlegm, sore throat.

People who indulge in sex and pregnant women should avoid haritaki.

As haritaki is a powerful drug, it is necessary that the drug be used under the close supervision of a qualified practitioner.

The seeds of haritaki are considered poisonous. They have to be carefully discarded while making the powder, etc. for medicinal use.

It is better to combine haritaki with the following rather than to consume it alone: Rock salt or black salt (during the months of June-July), sugar (August-September), dried ginger or *sonth* (October-November), long pepper (December-January), honey (February-March) and jaggery (April-May).

In Science

Beri, R. M. 1970. Phytosterol in some plant materials. *Indian Oil Soap J.* 35:274.

Grover, I. S. et al. 1992. Anti-mutagenic activity of *Terminalia chebula* (Myrobalan) in *Salmonella typhimurium. Indian J. Exp. Biol.* 30(4):339–41.

Howes, F. N. 1953. *Vegetable Tanning Materials.* London: Butterworths Scientific Publications.

Haslam, E. 1966. *Chemistry of Vegetable Tannins.* London & New York: Academic Press.

Hussein–Ayoub, S. M. and L. K. Yankov. 1985. Algicidal properties of tannins. *Filoterapia* 56(4):227. (Tannin fights germs.)

———— 1985. On the molluscicidal activity of the plant phenolics. *Filoterapia* 56(4):225.

Inamdar, M. C. and M. R. Rajarama Rao. 1962. Studies on the pharmacology of *Terminalia chebula*. *J. Scient. Ind. Res.* 21C:345. (Antispasmodic.)

Kannan, L. V. et al. 1960. Estimation of tannins in myrobalan (*Terminalia chebula* Retz.). *Indian J. Pharm.* 22:314–315.

Khalique, A. and M. Nizamuddin. 1972. Examination of *Terminalia chebula* I. Constituents of the fruit. *Bangladesh. Biol. Agric Soc.* 1:59.

Meera, P. et al. 1999. Antibacterial effect of selected medicinal plants on the bacteria isolated from fruit juices. *Geobios.* 26:17–20. (Of the 50 plants tested here, haritaki and pomegranate exhibit a high degree of antibacterial properties.)

Miglani, B. D. and A. S. Chawla. 1974. Chemical investigation of *Terminalia chebula*. *J. Inst. Chem.* 46:189.

Saxena, A. P. and K. M. Vyas. 1986. Antimicrobial activity of seeds of some ethnomedicinal plants. *J. Econ. & Taxon. Botany* 8:291–299. (Haritaki seeds show antibacterial activity.)

Sairam, T. V. 1997. Haritaki-Mother Superior. *Dignity Dialogue*. July.

Srivastava, J. C. and A. R. Verma. 1967. Chemistry of fruits of *Terminalia chebula*. *Indian Agric.* 11:69.

Tripathi, V. N. et al. 1983. Clinical Trial of *Haritaki* (*Terminalia chebula*) in treatment of simple constipation. *Sachitra Ayurved* 35 (11):737–40.

39

Gokhru

Tribulus terrestris

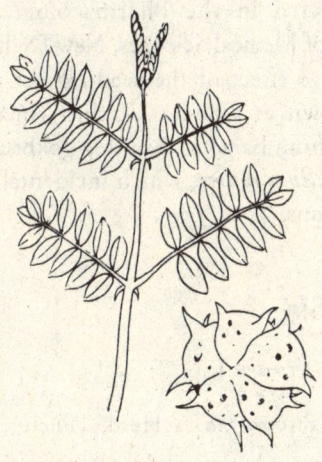

The Erotic Queen

—A Tamil name for gokhru

One of the Ten Great Roots

Appearances can be deceptive. Gokhru, an ugly and thorny weed often found in wastelands, like a municipality, controls the sewage disposal system inside the human body. It assists in the prompt elimination of toxin, stones, etc. that clog the genito-urinary tract.

Gokhru is one of the Ten Great Roots that constitute the popular Ayurvedic preparation, Dasamula. Apart from the root, the fruit and the whole plant also exhibit pharmacological action. The fruit is reported to be beneficial in curing sexual debility, as it enhances semen quality.

A chemical analysis of the fruit shows the presence of a fixed oil, sterols, resins, tannins, alkaloids and potassium.

Gokhru is diuretic. Its diuretic action is ascribed to the alkaloid fraction besides the potassium content.

In an experiment conducted in the Indian Institute of Panchakarma, Cheruthuruthy, the alcoholic extract of the fruits showed antibacterial action against *E. coli* and antifungal action against several fungal pathogens including *Candida albicans*. In yet another experiment conducted in the Pharmacological Research Unit, All India Institute of Medical Sciences, New Delhi, scientists recorded the hypotensive effect of the seed extract.

Tribulus terrestris is also known as Chhota Gokhru (small gokhru) in order to distinguish it from Bara Gokhru (big gokhru), a plant botanically known as *Pedalium murex,* which incidentally has identical medicinal applications.

Profile

Botanical Name	:	*Tribulus terrestris* L.
English Name	:	Land Caltrops, Goat's Head, Puncture Vine.
Indian Names	:	Bengali, Gujarati, Marathi, Punjabi : *Gokhru*
		Hindi : *Gokhru, Chhota Gokhru*
		Kannada : *Negalu, Senna Negalu*
		Malayalam : *Nerinnil*
		Marwari : *Kanti*
		Sanskrit : *Gokshura, Shvadamstra, Laghu Gokshura*
		Tamil : *Nerunjil, Kamarasi*
		Telugu : *Palleru*
		Ayurvedic : *Gokshura*

	Unani	: *Gokharu khurd.*
Chinese Name	:	*Chi li.* Family Zygophyllaceae.
Appearance	:	A thorny creeper. The thorns resemble the horns of cattle. Flowers, yellow, solitary with 4 petals. Fruit, 5-angled, covered with two types of spines—large and small. The plant has the smell of sugar cane.
Distribution	:	Grows wild throughout India and also in other tropical and warm temperate regions, upto 1000m.
Medicinal Parts	:	Fruit, the whole plant, root.
Preparations	:	Powder (500mg to 1g dosage), decoction, medicated oil.
Ayurvedic Preparations	:	*Dasamularishtam, Brihatyadi Kashayam, Himasagara Tailam, Vastyamayantaka Ghritam, Gokshuradi Avelaha, Gokshuradi Churan, Gokshuradi Guggal.*
Unani preparations	:	*Ma'zun Zanjibil, Lubab-al-Asrar, Sharbat Mudir, Sufuf Kalan, Sharbat Bazuri Motadil.*

In Tradition

AILMENT	PRESCRIPTION
❧ Sexual debility in men	: Boil a pinch of gokshura powder and ashwagandha powder in 1 cup milk and drink at bedtime for 10 days.

: Crush a whole plant including the fruit and soak in 1 cup goat's milk for three hours. Grind the plant with a little water and filter. Add 1 tsp honey and drink.

: Crush a whole plant with the fruit and boil along with 2 tsp each dried ginger, black pepper and long pepper; 1 tsp each cloves, bamboo-rice and 1 pinch of nutmeg powder in 4 cups water. Take $1/2$ cup twice daily for a week.

❧ Backache : Boil a pinch of gokshura and $1/4$ tsp dried ginger in 1 cup milk and drink. (*Note:* External application of ginger paste and eucalyptus oil may also be necessary.)

❧ Blockage of urine flow, leucorrhoea : Make a porridge with the following: 1 cup rice and 1 tsp each powder of gokshura fruit and root. Add a little sugar and drink for a few days.

❧ Blockage of urine flow, burning sensation during urination : Boil in 3 cups water 1 tsp crushed fruit and $1/2$ tsp coriander seeds till the volume is reduced to half. Take 2 tbsp twice daily for a few days.

❧ Blood in urine : Thoroughly wash the whole plant along with the root system. Extract $1/4$ cup juice. Mix in 1 cup of milk or buttermilk. Drink daily for a week.

❧ Body-heat, burning sensation in the eyes, urine retention, watery eyes : Boil in 4 cups water one cleaned plant each of gokhru and durva (*Cynodon dactylon*) after crushing them till the volume is reduced to 1 cup. Filter and drink $1/2$ cup thrice daily for 3 days.

✦ Jaundice,
urinary ailments

: Grind a whole plant along with the fruit into a very fine powder with 1 tsp cinnamon, 5 cardamoms and $1/2$ cup sugar candy. *Dose:* $1/2$ tsp along with water thrice daily before meals.

✦ Leucorrhoea,
venereal diseases

: Wash thoroughly one whole plant, with root system, flowers, fruits, etc. and also a whole plant of *bhumyamlaki.* Grind them into a very fine paste. Take 1 tbsp along with 1 cup curd twice daily for a week.

Note: Individual results may vary.

In Science

Bose, B. C. et al. 1963. Some aspects of chemical and pharmacological studies of *Tribulus terrestris. Indian J. Med. Sci. 17:291.* (The diuretic action may be ascribed to the alkaloid fraction besides the potassium content.)

Chakraborty, B. and N. C. Neogi. 1978. Pharmacological properties *of Tribulus terrestris* Linn. *Indian J.Pharm. Sci.* 40(2):50–52. (The alcoholic extract of the fruit produced CNS stimulant property, characterized by restlessness in experimental rats.)

Chopra, R. N. et al. 1956. *Glossary of Indian Medicinal Plants.* New Delhi: CSIR. (Gokshura's properties and uses: diuretic, cooling, tonic, aphrodisiac, in painful micturition, calculus affections, urinary discharges and impotence, in gout and kidney related diseases.)

Dipak, P. et al. 1985. *Evaluation of Tribulus terrestris (Chotagokhare). Indian Drugs.* 22(6):332–333. (Analgesic role of the drug.)

Harvey, S. K. 1966. Preliminary experimental study of the diuretic activity of some indigenous drugs. *Indian J. Med. Res.* 54(8):774–778. (Gokshura's contribution.)

Jaytilak, P. G. et al. 1976. Effect of an indigenous drug (Speman) on accessory reproductive functions of mice. *Indian J. Exptl. Biol.* 14(2):170–173. (The drug possessed anabolic and androgen-like activity.)

Joshi, C. G and N. G. Nagar 1952. Antibiotic activity of some Indian medicinal plants. *J. Sci. Industr. Res.* 11B(6):261. (Fruit exhibited activity against *S. aureus and E. coli*)

Mahato, S. B. et al. 1978. Screening of *Tribulus terrestris* plant for diosgenin. *J. Instn. Chem. India.* 50:49.

———. 1981. Steroidal glycosides of *Tribulus terrestris. J. Chem. Soc. Perkin Trans.* 1:2405.

Mehta, A. P. et al. 1982. Clinical trial of stonone in the management of urolithiasis and crystalluria. *J. Sci. Res. Plants Med.* 3 (2 and 3):61–63. (Stonone, a compound preparation administered to patients at a dosage of 2 tablets twice a day for 10 to 21 days was found effective without any side effects.)

Misra, D. N. and G. D. Shukla. 1984. Mustong in sexual inadequacy— clinical trial. *Nagarjun* 28(3):7–9. (2 tablets of Mustong containing the drug and 5 other plants taken at bedtime for a week increased sexual desire in patients without side effects.)

Nag, T. S. et al. 1979. Phyto-chemical studies of *Tribulus alatus.* Tribulus *terrestris* and *Agave wightii:* Contents of primary and secondary products. *Comp. Physiol. Ecol.* 4:157.

Sharma, H. C. and J. L. Narula. 1978. Chemical investigations of flowers of *Tribulus terrestris. Chem. Era.*13:15; Chem. Abstr. 1978, 88:19055k.

Sharma, K. and A. S. Puri, 1976. Ayurvedic treatment of Polycythaemia (Case report). *J. Res. Indian Med. Yoga and Homoeo.* 11(1):117–118. (A compound preparation containing gokshura and other herbs brough the blood profile to normal levels.)

Singh, R. C. P. and C. S. Sisodia. 1971. Effect of *Tribulus terrestris* fruit extracts on chloride and creatinine renal clearance in dogs. *Indian J. Physiol. Pharmacol.* 15:93–96. (Ether extract of fruit caused diuresis.)

Unikashvili, R. S. 1972. Histochemical characteristics of liver in experimental hypercholesterolemia under the action of *Tribulus terrestris* saponins. *Soobsheh. Akad. Nauk. Gruz. SSR.* 67(3):729–731, *Chem. Abstr. 78:12203.* Saponin found effective.

40

Ashwagandha
Withania somnifera

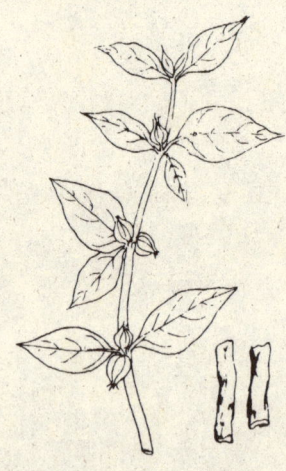

Ashwagandha, the rejuvenator

—Dhanvantari Nighantu

The Plant that Smells of Horses!

The leaves, roots and fruits of ashwagandha have long been used as medicine. The Sanskrit name of the plant refers to the peculiar odour of the root—an odour somewhat akin to that of a stable full of horses! The drug is also believed to impart the fabled sexual energy of the horse.

Ashwagandha is to the Indians what ginseng is to the Chinese: a tonic that imparts strength to the weak and cures impotence. Unfortunately, the world which has glorified ginseng has yet to wake up to ashwagandha!

However, the drug has become increasingly popular. Till recently the domestic need of this drug was met from the wild growth of this plant in the Bikaner, Nagaur and Pilani areas of Rajasthan. Most of the roots now available in various markets are obtained from cultivated plants, which are reported to differ from the wild ones in their therapeutical action, though the alkaloids present are the same. In view of these differences, some botanists consider the cultivated plant distinct from the wild one and have given it a new specific name: *Withania ashwagandha!*

The Root

The root facilitates conception. Scientific experiments have endorsed its antibacterial property. Its role in the treatment of ulcers, cough, rheumatism, leucoderma, etc. has now been fairly well established.

The Leaf

The leaf finds its use in the treatment of tumours and tuberculous glands. In folk medicine the leaf decoction is administered to young mothers to increase the milk outflow.

The Fruit

The fruit has an analgesic, diuretic, proteolytic and sedative action.

The importance of ashwagandha in Indian medicine can be gauged by the fact that over 100 drug preparations with ashwagandha as a major ingredient are available both in the Ayurvedic and Unani systems of medicine.

Profile

Botanical Name	:	*Withania somnifera* (L) Dunal.
English Name	:	Winter Cherry.
Indian Names	:	Bengali,
		Hindi,
		Marathi : *Askandhatilli*
		Punjabi : *Asgandh, Ashwagandha*
		Gujarati : *Asan, Asor, Ghoda, Asor*
		Kannada : *Hiremaddinegida Kiremallinagida, Asvagandhi*
		Malayalam : *Amukkiram, Pevetti*
		Sanskrit : *Ashwagandha, Varahakarmi, Turangigandha*
		Tamil : *Amukkiran Kizhangu*
		Telugu : *Pillivendramu, Asvagandi.*
Family	:	Solanaceae.
Appearance	:	Erect, evergreen, hairy shrub. Roots, stout, fleshy, whitish-brown. Leaves, simple, egg-shaped. Flowers, inconspicous, light green or pale yellow, in clusters. Fruits, berries, small, orange-red when mature, enclosed by the enlarged calyx. Seeds, many, kidney-shaped, yellow.
Distribution	:	Found throughout the drier parts of India in the wastelands. Also cultivated in Rajasthan.
Medicinal Parts	:	Root, leaf.
Medicinal Preparations	·	Powder, decoction, medicated ghee.
Ayurvedic Preparations	:	*Ashwagandharishtam, Chyavanpraasam, Valiya-Narayana Tailam.*

In Tradition

AILMENT	PRESCRIPTION

❧ Boils, inflammation : Pluck the fresh leaves of the plant and use as bandage.

❧ Carbuncle, inflammation, etc. : Spread a little castor oil on the leaf-surface and heat slightly over a naked flame. Apply a few such leaves on the affected areas.

❧ Cold, cough, gynaecological disorders, phlegm, watery nose : Mix $1/2$ tsp root-milk powder in honey and lick slowly once or twice a day.

: Mix $1/2$ tsp root-milk powder in warm water and drink once or twice a day.

❧ Conjunctivitis : Use pure leaf juice as eye drops.

❧ Fatigue, loss of appetite, obesity : Take $1/2$ tsp root-milk powder (See recipe below) with 1 tsp honey or 1 cup milk twice daily.

❧ Fatigue, spermatorrhoea : Mix $1/2$ tsp root-milk powder in a cup of warm milk and drink twice a day.

❧ Female gynaecolo-gical disorders, haemophilia, lumbago, sterility, disorders, etc. : Mix $1/2$ tsp root-milk powder with equal quantities of sugar, honey, powder of long pepper and ghee. Take once or twice a day.

✤ Female sterility, nervous weakness, physical weakness, sexual debility : Mix 1/2 tsp root-milk powder along with 1 tbsp palm sugar, in 1 cup cow's milk. Take at bedtime.

✤ Fever : Soak 5 tbsp leaves in a pot of water. Substitute this for your drinking water.

✤ Giddiness, palpitation of the heart : Mix 1/2 tsp root-milk powder in 1 tsp honey or 1 cup milk and drink.

✤ Glandular swellings caused by bubonic plague : Apply a paste of the root on the affected areas.

✤ Inflammation : Grind the rootstock and dried ginger along with a little hot water. Apply the paste over the affected areas.

✤ Involuntary ejaculation : Mix 1/2 tsp root-milk powder in a teaspoonful of ghee and eat twice a day.

✤ Joint pain, muscular pain : Boil 1 tbsp dried and powdered in 5 tbsp gingelly oil and apply on the affected parts when bearably hot.

✤ Lactation, to increase : Boil 1/2 tsp root-milk powder in 1 cup cow's milk. Drink twice daily.

✤ Pulmonary tuberculosis : Take 1/4 tsp root-milk powder with a glass of milk or water.

✤ Scrofula, toothache : Boil 1/2 tsp root-milk powder in 1 1/2 cup water. Add 1 teaspoonful each powdered long pepper and honey. Drink twice a day.

✤ Scrofula, tumour : Apply a paste of the leaves locally.

❧ Sexual debility   : Take $1/2$ tsp root-milk powder along with 1 tsp ghee twice daily.

❧ Ulcers,   : Dust the finely powdered root locally
   inflammation   on the affected areas.

Note: Individual results may vary.

A Word of Caution

Consumption of ashwagandha may result in increased body weight and hence those who are prone to obesity should use it in moderation. To increase body weight, boil $1/2$ tsp powder in 1 cup milk and drink twice a day.

Ashwagandha Root-Milk Powder

Ashwagandha root is often boiled in milk and then dried in the shade. When completely dry it is ground into a very fine powder. This powder is usually administered orally.

Ashwagandha Jam: A Health Tonic

Mix into 1 litre of amla juice, 1 tbsp each of the finely powdered roots of ashwagandha, liquorice and dried ginger. Add 4 tbsp each finely powdered long pepper and raisins, and 1 cup sugar. Boil this mixture over a low flame till it acquires a jam-like consistency. Bottle after cooling. A teaspoonful of this once a day is the recommended dose as a general health tonic.

In Science

Ahumada, F. et al. 1990. *Withania somnifera* extract. Its effect on arterial blood pressure in anaesthetized dogs. *Phytotherapy Res.* 5(3):111–114. (Controls blood pressure.)

Anbalagan, K. and J. Siddique. 1981. Influence of an Indian medicine (*Ashwagandha*) on acute phase reactants in inflammation. *Indian J. Exp. Biol. 19*:245.(Quells the swelling.)

————. 1985. *Withania somnifera* (*Ashwagandha*), a rejuvenating herbal drug which controls alpha-2-macroglobulin synthesis during inflammation. *Int. J. Crude Drug Res. 23(4)*:177–183. (Anti-inflammatory.)

Arora, R. B. and P. M. Stephen. 1959. Recent advances in pharmacology (1958–59) *Ann. Rev. Biochem. Res. India* 30:59–102. (Neuro pharmacological properties.)

Atal, C. K. et al. 1975. Pharmacognosy and Phytochemistry of *Withania somnifera. Lloydia 26*:238.

Babbar, O. P. et al. 1982. Evaluation of plants for anti-viral activity. *Indian J. Med. Res.* 76 (Suppl.):54–65. (Exterminates *Ranikhet* and *Vaccinia* viruses.)

Badhwar, R. L. et al. 1946. Reputed abortifacient plants of India. *Indian J. Agri. Sci.* 16:342–355. (In Sindh and Punjab, the root of ashwagandha is occasionally used to effect criminal abortion.)

Bhatnagar, S. S. et al. 1961. Biological activity of Indian medicinal plants. Part I. Antibacterial, anti-tubercular and antifungal action. *Indian J. Med. Res.* 49(5):799–813. (The leaves fight against gram positive bacteria and a fungus, *Helminthosporium sativum.*)

Chakrabarti, S. K. et al. 1974. Variations in the anti-tumor constituents of *Withania somnifera. Experientia* 30 (8):852. (In cancer research.)

Chandra, V. et al. 1970. Studies on alkaloid bearing plants- I. *Withania somnifera* Dunal. *Indian Drugs Pharm. Ind.* 40:1–7.

Chaudhary, K. and R. K. Neogy. 1975. Mode of action of Withaferin A and Withanolide D. *Biochem. Pharmacol.* 24(8):919–920.

Chopra, R. N. et al. 1956. *Glossary of Indian Medicinal Plants.* New Delhi: Council of Scientific and Industrial Research. (Abortifacient and purgative properties of roots; coagulant property of seeds in milk.)

Das, P. K. et al. 1965. Cardiotonic activity of *ashwagandha* and ashwagandhinine, two alkaloids from *Withania somnifera. Biol. Abstr.* 46(20):7172; *Chem. Abstr.* 89127. (Effects on the cardiovascular system.)

Dey, A. C. 1964. *Folklore of Medicinal Plants of the Bhagirathi Valley (Himalayas).* Kandy, Ceylon. Proceedings of the International Symposium on Medicinal Plants. 7–20. (Root paste cures the glandular swellings of bubonic plague.)

Dey, P. K. and B. K. Chatterjee. 1968. Studies on the medicinal plants. *J. Res. Indian Med.* 3(1):9–18; *Biol. Abstr.* 51:72610, 1970. (Effects on neuro-pharmacological disorders.)

Dhar, M. L. et al. 1968. Screening of Indian plants for biological activity. Part I. *Indian J. Exptl. Biol.* 6(4):232–247. Effects on the cardiovascular system.)

Dhawan, B. N. et al. 1980. Screening of Indian plants for biological activity. Part IX. *Indian J. Exptl. Biol.* 18(6):594–606. (Further research on the cardiovascular system.)

Fontaine, R. and A. Vrdos. 1976. On the effect of different *Withania* extracts after oral applications to animals. *Planta Med.* 30(3):242–250. (On neuro-pharmacological disorders.)

Gandhi, A. et al. 1994. A Comparative pharmacological investigation of Ashwagandha and Ginseng. *J. Ethnopharmaco.* 44(3):131–135. (Ashwagandha, the Indian Ginseng.)

Gandhi, R. and B. L. Kaul. 1984. Studies on the anti-irradiation activity of *Ashwagandha. Stud. Biophys.* 103:37–40.

Garg, L. C. and G. C. Parasar. 1965. Effect of *Withania somnifera* on reproduction in mice. *Planta Med.* 13(1):46–47. (On the reproductive system.)

Gupta, O. P. et al. 1977. Pharmacological investigations of *Withania somnifera. Indian J. Pharm.* 39(6):163. (Oral administration of root extract of ashwagandha for 2 to 3 weeks exhibited adaptogenic property.)

Jamwal, K. S. and K. K. Anand. 1962. Preliminary screening of some reputed abortifacient indigenous plants. *Indian J. Pharm.* 24(9):218–220. (On the reproductive system.)

Jayaram, S. et al. 1993. Valuation of efficacy of a preparation containing combination of Indian medicinal plants in patients of generalised weakness. *Indian Drugs* 30(10):498–500.

Koman, M. C. 1918. *Aswagandha, Paramgyathi Churnam.* Report on the investigation of indigenous drugs. First Rep. 1918.

Kuppurajan, K. et al. 1980. Effect of *Aswagandha (Withania)* on the process of ageing in human volunteers. *J. Res. Ayur. Sid.* 1:247–258. (Significant increase in haemoglobin, RBC, hair melanin and seated stature.)

Kurup, P. A. 1956. Antibiotic principles of leaves of *Withania somnifera Curr. Sci.* 25:57.

Kurup, P. A. 1958. The antibiotic principles of *Withania somnifera.* Isolation of antibacterial activity. *Antibiotic Chemotherapy* 8:511.

Lakkar, S. 1981. Clinical trial of Rumalaya in osteoarthritis of knee. *Med. & Sur.* 21(8):21–23. (Clinical trial of Rumalaya in osteoarthritis of the knee-joint responded excellently in 61% of the patients.)

Majumdar, D. N. 1955. *Withania somnifera* Dunal. 11. Alkaloidal constituents and their chemical characterization. *Indian J. Pharm.* 17:158.

Malhotra, C. L. et al. 1961. Studies on *Withania somnifera.* Part III. The effect of total extract on the cardiovascualr system and respiration. *Indian J. Med. Res.* 49(3):448–460.

———. 1962. Effect of total alkaloids *Withania ashwagandha* on smooth muscles. *Indian J. Physiol. Pharmacol.* 6(2):24. (Howers blood pressure in dogs.)

———. 1965. Studies on *Withania somnifera* IV. Effect of total extract on smooth muscles. *Indian J. Physiol. Pharmacol.* 9(1):9–15. (Brings down high blood pressure.)

Mardikar, B. R. and K. A. Narendranath. 1984 Beneficial effects of herbs and their combination with breast-milk. *J. Nat. Integ. Med. Ass.* 26(8):221–224. (Seeds show coagulant property in milk.)

Misra, D. N. and G. D. Shukla. 1984. Mustong in sexual inadequacy—a clinical trial. *Nagarjun* 28(3):7–9.

Moza, P. N. et al. 1967. A simple method for estimation of total alkaloids in *Ashwagandha*. *J. Res. Indian Med.* 2:77–78.

Panda, S. and A. Kar. 1998. Changes in thyroid hormone concentrations after administration of Ashwagandha root extract to adult male mice. *J. Pharm. Pharmacology,* 50: 1065–1068. (Ashwagandha root extract enhanced the level of circulating thyroid hormones; the findings suggests that the plant extract primarily stimulated thyroid gland to synthesize or secrete thyrotoxine.)

Rai, N. P. et al. 1983. Experimental studies on an indigenous drug *Withania somnifera* Dunal in electrical-induced convulsions in albino rats. *Nagarjun* 26(9):206–208.

Rajyalaxmi, E. 1982. Observations on the effect of Lukol in post-I.U.D. leuorrhoea and bleeding. *Probe* 22(1):35–36. (Lukol, containing ashwagandha, cured 80% of the cases of leucorrhoea and the disease did not recur for a longer period.)

Sairam, T. V. 1997. Ashwagandha—The Indian Ginseng—*Dignity Dialogue* 2(9): 41–47.

Sahni, Y. P. and D. N. Srivastava. 1990. *Withania somnifera*: An indigenous anti-ulcerogenic drug. *Indian J. Indig. Medicine* 10(1):53–56. (Cures ulcers.)

Saxena, V. K. 1973. Anti-fertility agents of plant origin. *J. Res. Indian Med.* 8(3):79–86. (Effect on the reproductive system.)

Schwarling, A. E. et al. 1963. The alkaloids of *Withania somnifera*. *Lloydia* 26:238.

Sharma, A. K. and R. H. Singh. 1980. Screening of anti-inflammatory activity of certain indigenous drugs on carrageen in induced hind paw oedema in rats. *Bull. Medico-Ethno-Bot. Res.* 1(2):262–271. (Anti-inflammatory action noted.)

Shaw, B. P. and L. N. Maithy. 1982. Comparative study of certain Ayurvedic drugs on *Amlapitta*. *Nagarjun* 36(4):73–75. (Combination of yashtimadhu and ashwagandha during a clinical trial of 91 patients suffering from gastritis, acidity and ulcer resulted in comparatively more improvement and reqistered the least untoward side effects.)

Shohat, B. et al. 1970. Effect of Withaferin on Ehrlich ascites tumour cells and cytological observations. *Int. J. Cancer* 5(2):244–252; *Biol. Abstr.* 51:79324. (Use in carcinoma.)

Shukla, S. P. 1981. Anti-anxiety agents of plant origin. *Probe* 20(3):201–208. (Improves mental function, increases body weight, reduces mental fatigue in rats.)

Singh, N. et al. 1978. Pharmacological investigation of some indigenous drugs of plant origin for evaluation of their antipyretic, analgesic and anti-inflammatory activities. *J. Res. Indian Med. Yoga & Homeo.* 13(2):58–62.

———. 1981. A new concept on the possible therapy of stress disease with adaptogens (anti-stress drugs) of indigenous plant origin. *Curr. Med. Practice* 23(1):50.

———. 1982. *Withania somnifera (Ashwagandha)*, a rejuvenating herbal drug which enhances survival under stress (an adaptogen). *Int. J. Crude Drug Res.* 20(1):29.

———. 1986. Prevention of Urethane-induced lung adenomas by *Withania somnifera* (L) Dunal in albino mice. *Int. Jour. Crude Drug Res.* 24(2):90–100. (Ashwagandha increases physiological endurance, protects the liver and prevents stress-ulcers—all these go to endorse its traditional use in Ayurveda as a vitalizer; it also holds out a hope for the treatment of many stress diseases like arterosclerosis, premature ageing, arthritis, diabetes, hypertension and malignancy.)

Singh, R. H. and P. C. Malaviya. 1978. Studies of the psychotropic effect of an indigenous rasayana drug *aswagandha (Withania somnifera* Dunal) Part I. *Jour. Res. Ind. Med. Yoga & Homoeop.* 13(1):15–24. (In the treatment of anxiety neurosis.)

Singh, R. H. et al. 1979. Studies on the psychotropic effect of an Indian indigenous drug *Ashwagandha (Withania somnifera)*. Part II. Experimental Studies. *J. Res. Indian Med. Yoga & Homeo.* 14(1):49–54.

————. 1982. A conceptual and clinical study on the scope of *medhya-rasayana* and *vajikarna* therapy in *manasaroga* with special reference to the anti-anxiety and anti-depressant activity of certain drugs. *J. Res. Edn. Indian Med.* 4 (3–4):9–20. (In the treatment of anxiety and depression.)

Singh, S. P. et al. 1977. A pharmacological evaluation of anti-pyretic, analgesic and anti-inflammatory activities of some indigenous drugs. *Indian J. Pharmacol.* 9(1):8. (Analgesic, anti-rheumatic, antipyretic and anti-inflammatory.)

————. 1977. *Search for effective anti-fertility agents from indigenous plant sources.* M. D. Pharmacology. Thesis. Lucknow. K. G. Med. Coll.

Srivastava, S. K. et al. 1960. Estimation of the total alkaloids of *Withania somnifera* Dunal. *Indian J. Pharm.* 22:94–95.

Sudhir, S. et al. 1986. Pharmacological studies of leaves of *Withania somnifera. Planta Med.* 1:61–63. (The leaf extract plays a protective role in inflammations and liver infections.)

Thejomoorthy, P. et al. 1986. Pharmacological evaluation of R-compound in *Amukkara-churnam* for anti-inflammatory activity. *Indian Vet.* J. 63(7):548–552.

Tomar, V. S. et al. 1984. Effect of 'Gerefort'—a herbal compound drug on anoxic stress tolerance in animals. *Indian Drugs* 21(6):233–235.

Uma Devi, P. et al. 1993. Anti-tumor and radio-sensitizing effects of *Withania somnifera* (Ashwagandha) on a transplantable mouse-tumour, Sarcoma-180. *Indian J. Exp. Biol.* 31(7):607–611. (Fights cancer.)

Verma, V. 1982. Effect of *Ashwagandha* in mice. *Indian Drugs.* 20:469–471.

Vidya Prabhu, M. et al. 1990. Neuro-pharmacological activity of *Withania somnifera. Filoterapia* 61(3):237–240. (Strengthens the intellect.)

Glossary of English Medical Terms

Abortifacient: Causing abortion.

Abscess: Local inflammation of body tissues with deep suppuration caused by bacteria, which destroy the cells in the centre of the area and leave a cavity filled with pus.

Adrenalin: Hormone secreted by adrenal glands, which are located near the kidney. It affects circulation and muscular action. Used in medicine as a stimulant.

Allergy: An abnormal response by the body to food or foreign matter.

Amenorrhoea: Delayed menstruation.

Amoebiasis: Infection caused by amoeba, a single-celled protozoan.

Amphetamine: Powerful synthetic stimulant.

Amylases: Enzymes capable of hydrolysing starch and carbohydrates.

Analgesic: Relieving pain.

Anthelmintic (also *anthelminthic*): Destroying intestinal worms.

Antiamoebic: Reducing and preventing the growth of amoeba.

Anticarcinogenic: Reducing and preventing cancer.

Antidote: A substance that counteracts poison.

Antiemetic: Preventing vomiting.

Antiepileptic: Preventing epilepsy.

Antifungal: Reducing and preventing the growth of fungus.

Antihypertensive: Lowering blood pressure.

Antimicrobial: Reducing and preventing the growth of microbes.

Antiprotozoal: Reducing and preventing the growth of protozoans eg., amoeba.

Antipyretic: Reducing fever.

Antiseptic: Reducing and preventing the growth of microbes.

Antitumour: Reducing and preventing the growth of tumours.

Antitussive: Relieving coughing.

Aphrodisiac: Exciting sexual activity.

Arrhythmia (also *arhythmia*): Abnormal rhythm of the heart-beat.

Arteriosclerosis: Hardening of arteries and other degenerative changes in them.

Artery: One of the vessels that convey blood from heart to the body.

Ascites: Fluid-retention in the peritoneal cavity of the abdomen.

Asthma: Periodic attacks of difficulty in breathing.

Bactericidal: Destroying bacteria.

Bacterium (pl. *bacteria*): Single-celled organism which brings about decay, disease, or builds up nitrogen compounds in the soil.

Bad Breath (also *halitosis*): Caused by poor dental hygeine, smoking, alcohol consumption, etc. Also a symptom of many disorders such as cancer of the mouth, throat, lungs, constipation, diabetes, gastritis, gingivitis, liver failure, sinusitis, underproduction of saliva, etc.

Bile: Thick, oily fluid excreted by the liver, helpful in digestion of fats.

Biliousness: Disorder of bile production (to excess).

Blood pressure, High: See Hypertension.

Blood pressure, Low: See Hypotension.

Blood: Fluid contained in arteries and veins of the body that carries nutrients to, and waste away, from all tissues. Made up of cells and plasma.

Bradycardia: Slow heart rate.

Bronchitis: An inflammation of the mucous lining of the bronchial tubes.

Carcinoma: Cancer, especially of epithelial origin.

Cardiac: Of the heart.

Cardio-vascular: Pertaining to the heart and the blood vessels.

Carminative: Expelling gas from the stomach and the intestine.

Cataract: Any opacity of the crystalline lens of the eye.

Cholera: Epidemic disease with violent vomiting and purging, cramps and collapse, endemic in India and epidemic elsewhere.

Cholesterol: Steroid alcohol present in animal cells and body fluids. Excess can lead to gallstones.

Colic: Acute abdominal griping pain caused by various abnormal conditions in the bowels.

Colitis: Inflammation of the colon.

Colon: The longest portion of the large intestine.

Compress: A lint or pad that is soaked in hot or cold substances and applied to the body for relief of swelling and pain.

Conjunctivitis: Inflammation of the transparent membrane covering the eyeball.

Constipation: Condition of bowels in which defecation is irregular and difficult.

Contraceptive: Preventing pregnancy.

Convulsion: Generalized involuntary spasm of the voluntary muscles.

Decoction: A herbal preparation, where the plant material (usually bark, roots, etc.) is boiled in water and reduced to make a concentrated extract.

Diabetes: Disease characterized by excessive discharge of glucose-containing urine, with thirst and emaciation, caused by the failure of pancreas to secrete an adequate amount of insulin and the resultant accumulation of glucose in the blood.

Diarrhoea: Excessive looseness of bowels.

Diuretic: Increasing the formation of urine.

Dropsy: Generalized accumulation of fluid in body; edema.

Dysentery: Disease with inflammation of mucous membrane and glands of large intestine, with mucous and bloody evacuations.

Dysmenorrhoea: Painful and difficult menstruation.

Dyspepsia: Indigestion or impaired digestion.

Dyspnea: Laboured breathing.

Dysuria (also *dysury*): Painful and difficult passage of urine.

Earache: Pain in ear, usually due to inflammation.

Eczema: An itching disease of the skin.

Elephantiasis: Tropical disease leading to huge swelling of the tissues especially in the lower limbs.

Emetic: Producing vomiting.

Emmenagogue: Stimulating or restoring menstrual flow.

Enzymes: Catalysts produced by living cells.

Eosinophil: Any cell which is stained readily with the dye eosin.

Eosinophilia: A pathological excess of eosinophils in blood.

Epilepsy: A nervous disorder, usually chronic, with characteristic convulsions of sudden onset, a tonic spasm often with crying and arrest of breathing followed by twitching, biting of tongue, frothing at the mouth, relaxation of the sphincter.

Epiphora: Continuous overflow of tears.

Epistaxis: Nosebleeds.

Erysipelas: Infection of the skin with *streptococci*.

Estrogen (also *oestrogen*): The generic term for female sex hormones.

Expectorant: Causing or stimulating expectoration to cough up and spit.

Fatigue: Exhaustion.

Febrifuge: Eliminating fever.

Fever: Elevation of body temperature.

Flatulence: Wind or gas in the stomach or intestine.

Flavanoids: Antioxidants which act on the immune system.

Fomentation: A hot compress.

Fungus: Mould.

Galactagogue: Increasing milk secretion.

Gastritis: Inflammation of the stomach.

Gastro-enteritis: Inflammation of the mucous membrane of the stomach and the intestine.

301

Giardiasis: Infestation of the intestinal tract with *Giardia lamblia*, a flagellate protozoan causing severe diarrhoea.

Glaucoma: A disease characterized by abnormally high pressure of the fluids within the eyeball, with consequent pain and impairment or loss of vision.

Goitre: Enlargement of the thyroid gland.

Gram-positive: Said of bacteria which stain when treated with methyl violet, followed by iodine and then by acetone or ethanol. Bacteria which do not stain are called gram-negative.

Haemoptysis: Spitting up of blood from the lungs.

Haemorrhage: Severe loss of blood from a blood vessel.

Haemorrhoids: Varicose dilatation of veins at the lower end of the rectum and the anus; piles.

Hematuria: The passing of blood in urine.

Hepatitis: A swelling and soreness of the liver.

Hernia: Protrusion of a viscus or part of a viscus, through an opening in the cavity containing it.

Hormone: A secretion from endocrine or ductless glands, exercising a stimulatory physiological action on other organs to which it is carried by the blood. Examples: thyroxin, adrenalin, corticosterone, insulin, oestradiol, etc. Such secretions are also formed in the actively growing parts of plants.

Hydrophobia: Aversion to water, especially as symptom of rabies; rabies.

Hypertension: High arterial pressure.

Hypoglycaemia: A below normal concentration of sugar in blood.

Hypotension: Low blood pressure; a fall in the blood pressure below the normal range.

Hysteria: A psychoneurosis, resulting from the conflict between the ego and the primitive tendencies of the id, in which the latter tendencies are repressed, and are thus excluded from the direct conscious expression, it being assumed that the unconscious, repressed material finds an indirect physical outlet through conversion, producing the hysterical symptoms.

Inflammation: The reaction of living tissue to injury or infection; swelling.

Insomnia: Chronic inability to sleep.

Ischaemia: A local, usually temporary deficiency of blood.

Itch (also *itching*): An irritating cutaneous disorder involving a persistent impulse to scratch.

Jaundice: Increase in bile pigments in blood.

Laxative: Promoting bowel movements.

Leprosy: Chronic, endemic bacterial disease caused by *Mycobacterium lepriae*, characterized by ulceration and thickening of the skin with loss of sensation and in severe cases, deformity and blindness.

Leucoderma: Depigmentation of the skin.

Leucorrhoea: An abnormal mucous discharge from the vagina.

Lipase: A fat-digesting enzyme.

Liver: An organ secreting bile which plays a key role in excretion.

Lumbago: Backache in the loin region.

Menorrhagia: Irregular profuse bleeding irrespective of menstrual cylce in women.

Migraine: A pathological headache, often on only one side, characterized by nausea and sensory disturbances.

Mouth ulcer: White or grey open sores with an outer ring of red inflammation, appearing inside of the lips, cheeks or on the floor of the mouth, caused by aggressive brushing of the teeth, ill-fitting dentures, accidental biting, etc.

Mucus: A thick, white liquid secreted by mucous glands.

Mumps: An acute infectious disease caused by a virus.

Myocardial infarction: Death of a part of the heart muscle, caused by a reduction or complete stoppage of blood supply.

Neurasthenia: A condition characterized by lack of physical and mental vigour, often by the presence of phobias.

Nocturnal emissions: Involuntary ejaculation of semen during sleep.

Obesity: A bodily condition in which there is an excess of fat in relation to other bodily components; presumed to exist when an individual is 20% or more over the normal weight.

Ophthalmia: An inflammation of the superficial tissue of the eye, especially of the conjunctiva.

Orchitis: Inflammation of the testicles.

Otitis media: Inflammation of the middle ear, caused often by the spread of throat infection.

Otitis: Inflammation of the ear.

Oxytocic: Stimulating contraction of the uterine muscle, accelerating childbirth.

Oxytocin: Hormone produced by the pituitary glands, stimulating muscles of uterus.

Pathogen: Anything capable of producing disease.

Pharmacology: The study of drugs.

Phlegm: Thick mucus from the respiratory tract.

Piles: Enlarged painful veins in the rectum or around the anus.

Pneumonia: A general disease in which the essential lesion is an inflammation of the spongy tissue of the lung.

Poultice: A soft mush prepared by various substances with oily or watery fluids.

Pox: Blisters and scars on the skin caused by certain diseases.

Psoriasis: Chronic skin-disease in which red, scaly patches develop.

Purgative: Relieving constipation.

Pus: The yellowish fluid formed by suppuration, consisting of serum, white blood cells, bacteria and the debris of tissue destruction.

Pustules: Pimples.

Pyorrhoea: A gum-infection.

Rejuvenation: The process of restoring vitality, especially the renewal of youthful, physiological vigour in the aged and senescent.

Rheumatism: Pain, swelling and deformity of joints of unknown cause.

Ringworm: A fungal infection.

Saponins: A group of glycosides, useful as detergents. Large doses of them in the blood-stream may prove fatal due to haemolysis (by dissolving the red blood corpuscles). Since they are feebly absorbed from the gastro-intestinal tract, their oral administration is, generally, without danger. They are mild laxatives, diuretics and expectorants.

Scabies: A skin-disease caused by a mite.

Sedative: Tending to soothe.

Sore: An ulcer or wound.

Spadix: A spike with a swollen, fleshy axis.

Spermatorrhoea: Frequent, involuntary discharge of semen, in the absence of sexual excitement or intercourse.

Spleen: A ductless gland situated at the left side of the cardiac end of the stomach.

Sterility: Inability to reproduce.

Steroids: Fat soluble organic compounds that occur naturally in flora and fauna and play many important functional roles.

Tachycardia: Excessive rapidity in the action of the heart.

Tannin: Widespread in plants, particularly in bark, leaves, etc. They prevent bacterial growth and thus aid in healing. By contracting blood-capillaries, tannins can help in preventing haemorrhages.

Throat: Area between the mouth and oesophagus.

Thyroid: Located below the larynx.

Tuberculosis (also *TB*): Caused by tubercle bacilli, it is an infectious disease, having varied manifestations in lung, bone or brain.

Ulcer: A slow-healing wound with superficial loss of tissue.

Urine: Excretion of kidneys, stored in the bladder and eliminated through urethra.

Vaso-dilating: Causing relaxation of blood vessels resulting in lowering of blood pressure.

Venereal sores: Diseases transmitted through coitus.

Vermifuge: Expelling worms from the intestine.

Virus: Minute organism that causes diseases such as common cold, chicken pox, smallpox, measles, mumps, poliomyelitis, etc.

Viscus: Any one of the organs situated within the chest and the abdomen: heart, lungs, liver, spleen, etc.

Vitamin: Any of the numerous substances, essential for nutrition, occuring naturally in food; also synthesized.

Vitamin A: Vital to good vision and is best obtained through natural sources. For instance, the pods of moringa are rich in B-carotene, which is converted into Vitamin A within the body. In the synthetic form, it has been proved to be toxic, particularly taken in large amounts.

Wheezing cough: Cough with whistling or piping sound.

Wound: An injury or break in the skin.

Glossary of Non-English Terms

Amlapitta: non-ulcer dyspepsia.

Ayurveda: 'The Veda of Life', the Indian system of medicine, as dealt with in the Atharva Veda.

Bhutas: spirits; elements.

Churan (also *Churanam, Churana*): powder.

Hakim (also, *Hakeem*): an Arabic word meaning a physician.

Kapha (also *Sleshma*): the bodily water humour; it implies the functions of heat regulation and also formation of various preservative fluids, e.g., mucus, synovia, etc.

Karappaan: eczema.

Kayakalpa: a treatment that arrests or retards the ageing process.

Medhya: a drug capable of improving the intellect and memory.

Panchakarma: five types of detoxification prescribed for healing.

Pitta: the bodily fire humour, which helps thermogenic and metabolic processes such as digestion, assimilation, tissue-building, endocrine activities, etc.

Rasam: a popular South Indian soup, made of lentils, tamarind, coriander seeds, cumin, asafoetida, curry leaves, etc.

Rasayana: a rejuvenative therapy or drug which regenerates body and mind, preventing decay and ageing.

Samhita: a part of the Vedic literature dealing with do's and dont's called *smriti*; in all, there are 18 Samhitas.

Sloka: a distich verse.

GLOSSARY OF NON-ENGLISH TERMS

Tantra: a system of worship.

Tapasya: severe religious austerity.

Trikatu: a mixture of dry ginger, black pepper and long pepper.

Triphala: a mixture of three myrobalans: emblic (amlaki), chebulic (haritaki) and beleric (bibhitaki).

Unani: conventional Arabian system of medicine.

Upanishad: mystical writing in Sanskrit aimed at exploring the Vedas; in all, there are over 100 Upanishads.

Vaid (also *Vaidya, Vaidyar, Baid*): one who is trained in medical science.

Vata (also *Vayu*): the bodily air humour, explaining all the biological phenomena, controlled by the central and autonomous nervous systems.

Vedas: the Hindu scriptures; in all, there are four vedas: Rig, Yajur, Sama and Atharva.

Vedic: pertaining to the Vedas.

Glossary of Plants and Other Ingredients

This glossary covers only those plants which are not discussed under a separate chapter in this book. Abbreviations used: (E)= English; (S)= Sanskrit; (H)=Hindi; (T)= Tamil.

Ajwain (H): *Trachyspermum ammi.* Omum (T). A herb with seed-like fruits used in cuisine as well as medicine.

Aniseeds (E): *Pimpinella anisum.* Saunf, Saurif (H). A herb with seed-like fruits yielding anise oil, which is used in medicine.

Anjir (H): *Ficus* carica. Fig (E). Fruits, a source of rich nutrition.

Asafoetida (E): *Ferula asafoetida.* Hing (H). Perungayam (T). An ideal wind-expeller from the digestive tract.

Ash-gourd (E): *Benincasa hispida.* A common vegetable in Indian cuisine. In Ayurveda, the fruit juice is administered as a specific in haemoptysis and other haemorrhages from the internal organs.

Asoka (also, Asokam): *Saraca asoca.* The bark has been widely used since time immemorial for the treatment of dysmenorrhoea, menorrhagia, uterine haemorrhages, etc. The tree is regarded as a symbol of love and is dedicated to Kama, the Indian God of Love.

Bamboo-rice (E): Grains of *Bambusa arundinacea.*

Bariara (H): *Sida acuta.* Prickly sida (E). Mayir maanikaam (T). A common herb whose stem-fibre is used for ropes and twines.

Bel (H): *Aegle marmelos.* Vilvam (T). A thorny tree whose leaves, flowers, fruits, bark and roots have medicinal value.

Ber (H): *Ziziphus jujuba.* Chinese Date, Jujube (E). Ilandai (T). A host of the lac insects.

Besan (H): Gram-flour. An ideal soap-substitute available readily in the Indian kitchen.

Betel leaf (E): *Piper betle.* Paan (H). Vetrilai (T). The plant is useful in alcoholism, cough, fever, halitosis, impotency, leprosy, rheumatism, etc.

Bhringaraja (S): *Eclipta prostrata.* Karisilanganni (T). Found effective in the treatment of infective hepatitits. Myocardial depressant and hypotensive effects recorded.

Bhumyamlaki (S): *Phyllanthus niruri..* Keezhanelli (T). Jungli Amli(H).

Bitter orange (E): *Citrus aurantium.* Khatta (H).

Black pepper (E): *Piper nigrum.* Kali mirch (H). Milagu (T). Stimulates thyroid glands.

Camphor (E): *Cinnamomum camphora.* Kapoor (H). Karpooram (T). Useful for local application on sprains, inflammations and rheumatic pains. Internally administered in certain types of diarrhoea or as a cardiac stimulant. Camphor is also obtained from another plant: *Ocimum kilimandscharum.*

Cardamom (E): *Elettaria cadamomum.* Elaichi (H). Elakkai (T). Stimulates heart and spleen.

Catmint (also *Catnip*) (E): *Nepeta cataria.* An aromatic, European herb found in Kashmir, whose leaves are chewed to relieve toothache.

Chillies (E): *Capsicum frutescens.* Mirch (H). Milagai (T). Rich in Vitamin C.

Cinnamon (E): *Cinnamomum zeylanicum.* Dalchini (H). Lavangapattai (T). Fights toxins.

Cissampelos pareira: False Pareira Root (E). Harjori (H). The roots are used in cough, diarrhoea, dysentery and urinary infections.

Coconut (E): *Cocos nucifera.* Nariel (H). Thengai (T). Exhibits a very significant antifungal activity.

Common milk edge (also *Milk-bush, Indian tree spurge.*) (E): *Euphorbia tirucalli.* Thohar (H). Succulent spineless xerophyte with pencil-like branches and milky exudate; the roots are used as a fish-poison.

Copra (E): dried coconut fruit. *Cocos nucifera.*

Country mallow (E): Indian abutilon. *Abutilon indicum.* Kanghi(H).

Thuthi (T). Known in Ayurveda as *atibala*, the root is reportedly aphrodisiac.

Cucumber (E): *Cucumis sativus.* Khira (H). Vellari (T). A hairy climber with simple leaves. Its fruits are useful in vitiated conditions of *pitta*, burning sensation, fever, general debility, insomnia, jaundice, etc.

Cumin (E): *Cuminum cyminum.* Zeera (H). Jeeragam (T). Charaka Samhita says: 'Grind cumin seeds with a drop of ghee and a pinch of salt; apply for scorpion sting.'

Dhatura (H): *Datura stramonium.*

Dry ginger (E): Dried rootstocks of ginger, *Zingiber officinale.* Sonth (H). Chukku (T). One of the three ingredients in trekatu.

Fennel: *Foeniculum vulgare.* Saunf (H). An excellent stomach and intestinal remedy.

Fenugreek (E): *Trigonella foenum-graecum.* Methi(H). Vendhiyam (T). A carminative and stimulant.

Fig (E): *Ficus carica.* Anjeer (H). Athi (T).'The best food that can be taken by those who are brought low by long sickness...'—Pliny, the Roman Naturalist.

Four-o-clock plant (E): *Mirabilis jalapa.* Gulabbas (H). Andhimalli (T). Fam: Nyctaginaceae. The powdered seeds are used in cosmetics; flowers, a traditional source of a crimson dye.

Garlic (E): *Allium sativum.* Lasan (H). Poondu (T). Fam. Liliaceae. The bactericidal effect of garlic oil is found to be 24 times greater than that of carbolic acid.

Ghee (H): Clarified butter from cow's or buffalo's milk. Old ghee (*ghritam*) finds it use as an ideal vehicle for many a herbal medicine.

Gingelly oil (E): A popular cooking oil obtained from the seeds of sesame, *Sesamum indicum.* Til-ka-tel (H). Nallennai (T).

Gulkand (H): A confection made of rose petals.

Indravalli (also *Jyotishmati*?): *Cardiospermun halicacabum.* Mudakathan (T). The plant exhibits sedative effect on CNS, significant analgesic, anti-spasmodic and vaso-depressant action.

Jaggery (E): Gur (H). Unrefined cane sugar. Often added to the herbal medicines as a cheap substitute for honey.

311

Kanjaankorai (also *Naai-tulasi*) (T): *Ocimum album*. Belonging to the family of basils, Labiatae.

Kantakari (H): *Solanum virginianum*. (Synonyms: *Solanum surattense, Solanum xanthocarpum*). Extensively used for expelling phlegm and in the treatment of asthma, bronchitis and cough.

Karisilanganni (T): *Eclipta prostrata*. Svetabhringaraja (S).

Keezhanelli (T): *Phyllanthus amarus*. Jungli amla (H). A single-drug remedy for jaundice.

Kurutaka (S): *Pergularia daemia*. Veliparuthi (T). The leaf juice is an expectorant and an emetic.

Kustha (also *Kuth*) (H): *Saussurea lappa*. Costus (E). The roots are used medicinally as a carminative, stimulant and tonic. Also used in controlling bronchial asthma. Kashmiris and Garhwalis use the root to preserve their woollens against bugs and termites.

Lesser galangal (E): *Alpinia officinarum*. Rasana (S). Arattai (T). Two anti-tumour principles have been isolated recently by Japanese scientists.

Lime (E): *Citrus aurantifolium*. Nimbu (H). Elumitchai (T). 'Lime adds beauty and prosperity to a house.'—Matsya Purana.

Madhunashini (also *Gurmar*): *Gymnema sylvestre*. The leaves suppress the sweet taste in the tongue.

Manathakkaali (T): *Solanum nigrum*. Black nightshade (E). Makoy (H). The plant is useful in vitiated conditions of tridosha, asthma, cough, dyspepsia, rheumatalgia, swelling, vomiting, etc.

Miers (E): *Tinospora cordifolia*. Gulancha (H). Seendhil (T). An aqueous extract of the stem is experimentally demonstrated to reduce blood pressure.

Neem (H): *Azadirachta indica*. Margosa (E). Vembu (T). Of late, the tree has attracted such scientific attention for its medicinal and environmental roles.

Palm sugar (also *palmyrah sugar*) (E): sugar obtained from the palm, *Borassus flabellifer*.

Pudina (H): *Mentha arvensis*. Fieldmint (E). One of the Three Great Mints, known in the Indian kitchen for its tangy chutney.

Punarnava: *Boerhavia diffusa.* Mukaratte (T). The root-ointment exhibits significant anti-inflammatory properties.

Siora (also, *Dahia, Khorus*) (H): *Streblus asper.* (Syn. *Epicarpurus orientalis.*)

Slaked lime (E): Calcium hydroxide, produced when caustic lime is mixed with water, releasing much heat. Chuna (H). Chunnambu (T).

Soap-nut (E): *Sapindus emarginatus.* Ritha (H). Cultivated in North India.

Symplocos paniculata: Lodh (H). A small tree found in the Himalayas from Assam to Kashmir.

Tail pepper (also *Cubebs*) (E): *Piper cubeba.* Kabaabchini (H). Valmilagu (T). Used in folk treatments for cystitis, it contains Cubebin, the urinary antiseptic.

Talispatri (also *Baichi, Bilangra, Kantai*) (H): *Flacourtia indica.* Governor's Plum, Ramontchi (E). The root is useful in biliousness, poisonous bites, rheumatism, urinary diseases, etc. The edible fruit is used in cases of jaundice and enlarged spleen.

Trikatu (S): The Three Pungents: dry ginger, black pepper and long pepper.

Tulsi (H): *Ocimum sanctum.* Holy basil (E). Tulasi (T). 'To be sought after and cherished.'—Puranas.

Turmeric (E): *Curcuma longa.* Haldi (H). Manjal (T). 'A paste can drive away all poisons from the body.'—Matsya Purana.

Turpeth (also *Indian jalap*) (E): *Operculina turpethum.* Nisoth, Pithori (H). Recent laboratory experiments involving albino rats have endorsed the folk-use of roots in the treatment of acute inflammation.

Uthamani (T): *Pergularia daemia.*

Vidanga (S): *Embelia ribes.* Baberang (H). Vayu-vidangam (T). Seeds are used in folk-remedies as anthelmintic. A teniacide, embelin has been isolated.

Vishnukaranti (S): *Evolvulus alsinoides.* A specific for all kinds of fevers.

Yashtimadhu (S): *Glycyrrhiza glabra.* Liquorice (E). Atimadhuram (T). Mainly used in bronchial troubles.

Index

Cobra's Saffron, *see* Nagakesara
Coccinia indica, see Kovai
Coccinia cordifolia, see Kovai
Coccinia grandi's, see Kovai
Cold,
    Aloe for, 41
    Arkh for, 93
    Ashwagandha for, 289
    Chirchita for, 10
    Galangal for, 51
    Nagakesara for, 201
    Tamarind for, 259
    Vasaka for, 30
Colic,
    Arkh for, 94
    Calamus for, 20
Commiphora mukul, see Guggul
Commiphora wightii, see Guggul
Common Basil, *see* Sweet Basil
Common Jasmine, *see* Jasmine
Complexion improvement, Peepul for, 165
Conessi, *see* Kutaja
Congelation of blood, Tamarind for, 259
Congestion in lungs, Durva for, 136
Conjunctivitis,
    Ashwagandha for, 289
    Banyan for, 158
Constipation,
    Aloe for, 41
    Brahmi for, 70
    Haritaki for, 275
    Indian Acalypha for, 4
    Indian Barberry for, 76
    Katurohini for, 228

Keezhanelli for, 222
Peepul for, 166
Rose for, 249
Senna for, 102
Sweet Basil for, 216
Tamarind for, 258–59
Convulsions,
    Aloe for, 41
    Katurohini for, 229
Corns, Henna for, 187
Cough,
    Aloe for, 41
    Arkh for, 93
    Ashwagandha for, 289
    Calamus for, 20
    Chirchita for, 10–11
    Drumstick for, 206
    Flame of the Forest for, 83
    Galangal for, 50–51
    Indian Birthwort for, 59–60
    Long Pepper for, 234
    Shatavari for, 64
    Tamarind for, 259
    Vasaka for, 30–32
    Vibhitaki for, 268
Cough in children,
    Brahmi for, 70–71
    Calamus for, 20
Covel, *see* Kovai
Cracks, Henna for burning sensation in, 186
Cracks in heels, Banyan for, 158
Cracks in nipples, Castor for, 242
Cracks in sole,
    Banyan for, 158
    Peepul for, 166
Curaçao Aloe, *see* Aloe

Java Galangal, *see* Galangal
Java Plum, *see* Jamun
Jilledu, *see* Arkh
Joints pain,
    Arkh for, 94
    Ashwagandha for, 290
    Carrot for, 144
    Drumstick for, 207
    Henna for, 189
    Tamarind for, 261
Jungli Amla, *see* Keezhanelli
Jungli Amli, *see* Keezhanelli
Justicia adhatoda, *see* Vasaka

Kaarattu, *see* Carrot
Kachoramu, *see* Galangal
Kadu, *see* Katurohini
Kadugrubani, *see* Katurohini
Kadugu-Rohini, *see* Katurohini
Kadukka, *see* Haritaki
Kadukkai, *see* Haritaki
Kaidonda, *see* Kovai
Kakracha, *see* Flame of the Forest
kalajam, *see* Jamun
Kalajan, *see* Galangal
Kali, *see* Flame of the Forest
Kali Kutki, *see* Katurohini
Kali Tulsi, *see* Sweet Basil
Kalinga, *see* Kutaja
Kalingam, *see* Kutaja
Kalingam, *see* Kutaja
Kalojam, *see* Jamun
Kamakasturi, *see* Sweet Basil
Kamarasi, *see* Gokhru
Kanduri, *see* Kovai
Kanti, *see* Gokhru
Kopha aggravation, Vasaka for, 32

Kapur Kanti, *see* Sweet Basil
Karakayi, *see* Haritaki
Karakka, *see* Haritaki
Karalakah, *see* Indian Birthowrt
Karalakam, *see* Indian Birthwort
Karchi, *see* Kutaja
Karitaki, *see* Haritaki
Kariyapolam, *see* Aloe
Karpuratulasi, *see* Sweet Basil
Karu, *see* Katurohini
Karuka, *see* Durva
Karukappulu, *see* Durva
Kasappuveppilai, *see* Kutaja
Kashmal, *see* Indian Barberry
Kataki, *see* Katurohini
Katalati, *see* Chirchita
Katavala, *see* Aloe
Kathi, *see* Galangal
Katki, *see* Katurohini
Katuko, *see* Katurohini
Katukarohini, *see* Katurohini
Katumurukku, *see* Flame of the forest
Katurohini, 226–30
Katvi, *see* Katurohini
Keezhaarnelli, *see* Keezhanelli
Keezhakkanelli, *see* Keezhanelli
Keezhanelli, 219–25
Kengen, *see* Nagakesara
Keora, *see* Kutaja
Kesaramu, *see* Nagakesara
Kewar, *see* Kutaja
Khakria, *see* Flame of the forest
Khakro, *see* Flame of the forest
Kherwa, *see* Kutaja
Khokali, *see* Indian Acalypha
Khokhali, *set*, Indian Acalypha

Vatah, see Banyan
Vatavriksham, see Banyan
Vattagam, see Peepul
Vayampu, see Calamus
Vebhudipatri, see Sweet Basil
Veila, see Nagakesara
Vekhand, see Calamus
Velleruku, see Arkh
Velutha champagam, see Nagakesara
Veluthapala, see Nagakesara
Venereal diseases,
    Banyan for, 161
    Durva for, 138
    Gokhru for, 283
    Mandukaparni for, 108
Venereal sores, Indian Acalypha
    for, 5
Venereal ulcers, Mandukaparni
    for, 108
Venkatalati, see Chirchita
Venpala, see Kutaja
Veppalai, see Kutaja
Vepudupachcha, see Sweet Basil
Vibeedagam, see Vibhitaki
Vibhita, see Vibhitaki
Vibhilaki, 266–71
Vibhitakamu, see Vibhitaki
Vibhdhi-Pachai, see Sweet Basil
Visaghni, see Indian Birthwort
Visavega, see Indian Birthwort
Vision blurring, Mandukaparni
    for, 107
Vision impairments, Mandukapar-
    ni for, 107
Vistarakupala, see Kutaja
Vitis quadrangularis, see Bone-
    Setter
Vomiting,

Banyan for, 161–62
Long Pepper for, 235
Rose for, 251
Vondelega, see Mandukaparni
Vritta Pushpa, see Rose

Watery eyes,
    Gokhru for, 282–83
    Jamun for, 152
Watery nose, Ashwagandha for,
    289
Watery sperm,
    Banyan for, 161
    Drumstick for, 206, 208
    Tamarind for, 263
Weak and spongy gums, Guggul
    for, 128
Weak heart, Rose for, 249
Weeping eczema, Henna for, 190
Whitlow,
    Arkh for, 96
    Castor for, 244
    Durva for, 139
    Haritaki for, 276
Wild Asparagus, *see* Shatavari
Wild Carrot, *see* Carrot
Winter Cherry, *see* Ashwagandha
Withania somnifera, see
    Ashwagandha
Wounds,
    Aloe for, 42–43
    Calamus for, 22
    Chirchita for, 12
    Drumstick for, 208
    Durva for, 137, 139
    Guggul for, 128
    Henna for, 190
    Indian Acalypha for, 6